28 Days to a Better You!

High-Fiber Diet Plan

Copyright © 2020 by Sarah Pierce

All Rights Reserved.

CONTENTS

INTRODUCTION 4

HIGH-FIBER DIET 4

FOODS TO AVOID 4

FOODS TO PREFER 4

INSOLUBLE FIBER 5

SOLUBLE FIBER 5

HEALTH BENEFITS 6

HEALTH RISKS 10

GROCERY LIST WEEK 1 16

MEAL PLAN WEEK 1 17

GREEN SMOOTHIE 18

BACON & EGGS 19

STRAWBERRY SMOOTHIE 20

AVOCADO CAPRESE TOAST 21

CHICKEN CAPRESE WRAPS 22

ARUGULA SALAD 23

PASTA SALAD 24

BROWN RICE WITH VEGETABLES 25

FRIED SALMON 26

BEEF SALAD 28

CHICKEN SOUP 29

GROCERY LIST WEEK 2 30

MEAL PLAN WEEK 2 31

BLUEBERRY SMOOTHIE 32

SCRAMBLED EGGS 33

BANANA PANCAKES 34

AVOCADO EGG SALAD 35

AVOCADO TUNA SALAD 36

TOMATO & HEARTS OF PALM SALAD 37

QUINOA BOWL 38

GROCERY LIST WEEK 3 39

MEAL PLAN WEEK 3 40

AVOCADO BANANA SMOOTHIE 41

FRUIT SALAD 42

VEGETABLE & HUMMUS SALAD 43

AVOCADO & CHICKEN SALAD 44

VEGGIE SOUP 45

AVOCADO SALAD 46

CHOPPED GRILLED VEGGIE SALAD 48

CHICKEN SPINACH SALAD 49

GROCERY LIST WEEK 4 50

MEAL PLAN WEEK 4 51

PIZZA ROLL UPS 52

GRILLED SALMON WITH BROWN RICE 53

BAKED POTATO & BEANS 54

INSTANT PIZZA 55

CHICKPEA SPINACH SALAD 56

BAKED SALMON 57

THE HIGH-FIBER DIET GUIDE

INTRODUCTION

HIGH-FIBER DIET

High fiber diet includes eating a well-balanced diet which is rich in fiber like vegetables (carrots, beets, broccoli, collard greens, spinach, artichokes, potatoes) fruits (bananas, oranges, apples, mangoes, strawberries, raspberries) beans & legumes (Navy, white, garbanzo, kidney, peas, or lentils are all healthy choices), Bread & grains (wheat, brown rice, wild rice, and barley) and nuts (Almonds, pistachios, or pumpkin and sunflower seeds). Fiber comes only from plants, so you will need to include plant sources in your diet to get enough fiber.

FOODS TO AVOID

Enriched white bread, rolls, biscuits, and muffins.

Waffles, French toast, and pancakes. White rice, noodles, pasta, and cooked potatoes (no skin). Plain crackers, Cooked cereals.

FOODS TO PREFER

Brown or wild rice, Whole grains, cracked grains, or whole wheat products, Kasha (buckwheat), Corn bread or corn meal, Graham crackers, Bran, Wheat germ, Nuts, Granola, Coconut, Dried fruit, Seeds.

Fortunately, increasing your fiber intake is relatively easy — simply integrate foods into your diet that have a high percentage of fiber per weight.

INSOLUBLE FIBER

Does not dissolve in water. It is the bulky fiber that helps to prevent constipation, and is found in whole grains, wheat cereals, and vegetables such as carrots, celery, and tomatoes.

SOLUBLE FIBER

Dissolves in water and helps control blood sugar levels and reduce cholesterol. Good sources include barley, oatmeal, beans, nuts, and fruits such as apples, berries, citrus fruits, and pears.

PREBIOTIC SOLUBLE FIBER

These are relatively newly discovered soluble plant fibers. The technical name for this fiber is inulin or fructan. When these soluble fibers are fermented by the good colon bacteria, some further significant health benefits have been shown to occur by research in many medical centers.

These fibers are found in asparagus, yams and other root vegetables such as chicory, garlic, onion, leeks and in smaller amounts in wheat. This research has shown the following:

- Increase in good and decrease in bad colon bacteria
- Increase calcium absorption and enhanced bone mass
- Enhanced immune system
- Appetite and weight control by changing the hormone appetite signals to the brain
- May decrease colon cancer incidence
- Reduce or correct a leaky colon

HEALTH BENEFITS

Fiber offers a healthy and effective way to stay regular. But that's not the only reason why we should be including more in our diets. Some of the benefits include:

SKIN HEALTH
When yeast and fungus are excreted through the skin, they can trigger outbreaks or acne. Eating fiber can flush toxins out of your body, improving the health and appearance of your skin.

LOWER CHOLESTROL LEVELS
Soluble fiber found in beans, oats, flaxseed and oat bran may help lower total blood cholesterol levels by lowering low-density lipoprotein, or bad cholesterol levels. Studies also have shown that high-fiber foods may have other heart-health benefits, such as reducing blood pressure and inflammation.

HEALTHY HEART
A high fiber intake can also reduce your risk for metabolic syndrome, a group of risk factors linked to coronary heart disease, diabetes, and stroke. Fiber can also help to lower blood pressure, reduce inflammation, improve levels of HDL cholesterol, and shed excess weight around the abdomen.

CONTROLLING SUGAR LEVELS
In people with diabetes, fibers can slow the absorption of sugar and help improve blood sugar levels. A healthy diet that includes insoluble fiber may also reduce the risk of developing type 2 diabetes.

WEIGHT LOSS

Fiber-rich foods not only fill you up faster and keep you satisfied longer, they also prevent your body from absorbing some of the calories in the foods you eat.

Another study found that people who doubled their fiber intake to the recommended amount knocked off between 90 and 130 calories from their daily intake.

High fiber diets are more filling and give a sense of fullness sooner than an animal and meat based diet does. In addition, the soluble prebiotic fibers have been shown to turn off the hunger hormones produced in the wall of the gut and to increase the hormones that give a sense of fullness.

New medical research has shown that the bacterial makeup in the colon in overweight people is abnormal to the extent that they manufacture and absorb almost twice the number of calories through the colon wall.

PREVENT CANCER

There is some research that suggests eating a high-fiber diet can help prevent colorectal cancer. In addition to the anti-cancer effects of fiber, the foods that contain it-like veggies and fruits-are also rich in antioxidants and phytochemicals that could further reduce your odds, notes Sheth.

CHOLESTROL & REDUCED TRIGLYCERIDES

The soluble fibers are the ones that will reduce cholesterol levels when used on a regular basis. Psyllium husk and prebiotic soluble fiber will also reduce cholesterol. They may also reduce the incidence of coronary heart disease. Oats, flax seeds and legumes or beans are the recommended fibers.

CONSTIPATION

If your fiber intake is generally low, try including more high-fiber foods like fruits, vegetables and whole grains in your diet. This will increase both your soluble and insoluble fiber intake and could help relieve your problem. It's best to do this gradually, as dramatically increasing your intake in a short period could cause unwanted side effects like pain, gas and bloating.

BOWEL REGULARITY

A high fiber diet promotes regularity with a softer, bulkier and regular stool pattern. This decreases the chance of hemorrhoids, diverticulosis and perhaps colon cancer.

IMPROVED SLEEP

A study just published in the Journal of Clinical Sleep Medicine compared the effects of different foods on slow-wave sleep. They found that when study participants ate the recommended diet, which included high-fiber foods low in saturated fat and sugar, they fell asleep faster and had longer periods of deeply restful sleep.

COLON POLYPS & CANCER

Considerable research suggests that high fiber diet may prevent colon cancer. Certainly it makes sense to increase regularity and so speed the movement of cancer causing carcinogens through the bowel. In addition, reducing a heavy meat diet reduces the bile flow from the liver in a favorable way. This, too, reduces the amount of carcinogens that reach and are manufactured in the colon. Finally, a high fiber diet, including prebiotic soluble fiber, increases the integrity and health of the wall of the colon.

BACTERIA & COLON FUNCTION

The colon finishes the digestive process. Hopefully, the waste products move through in a nice regular manner. Insoluble fibers help this process by retaining water and so producing a bulkier, softer stool, which is easy to pass.

Recent research has shown that there are over 1,000 species of bacteria with a total bacterial count ten times the number of cells in the body. These bacteria play a major role in keeping the colon wall itself healthy. In addition, these good bacteria produce a very strong immune system for the body. They significantly increase calcium absorption and bone density. They provide other documented benefits. It is the soluble fibers in the diet that are so effective in stimulating the growth of good colon bacteria.

HEALTH RISKS

TOO MUCH FIBER INTAKE

The recommended daily intake of fiber is 25 grams per day for women and 38 grams per day for men. However, some experts estimate as much as 95 percent of the population don't ingest this much fiber.

While it appears most people fall short of their recommended fiber intake, it's actually possible to have too much fiber, especially if you increase your fiber intake very quickly. Too much fiber can cause:

- **Abdominal pain**
- **Loose stools or diarrhea**
- **Constipation**
- **Temporary weight gain**
- **Intestinal blockage in people with Crohn's disease**
- **Reduced blood sugar levels**

Call your doctor right away if you're experiencing nausea, vomiting, a high fever, or a complete inability to pass gas or stool.

FIBER & GAS

Everyone has intestinal gas and that is a good thing. It means that bacteria, hopefully the good ones, are thriving. The normal amount of flatus passed each day depends on sex and what is eaten. The normal number of flatus is 10-20 times a day.

High-fiber diets are believed to cause bloating by increasing certain populations of healthy, fiber-digesting gut bacteria. They produce gas as a byproduct. These findings suggest that carbs and proteins change the gut bacteria population. Soluble fiber should always be used in a gradual manner. If too much is consumed at any one time, then excess, but harmless, intestinal gas can occur.

Prebiotic fibers tend to cause the production of short-chain fatty acids which acidify the colon. This, in turn, reduces or stops the growth of bacteria that make the smelly hydrogen sulfide gases that produce noxious flatus. People who consume many vegetables with prebiotics or take a prebiotic fiber supplement often have non-odoriferous flatus.

FIBER & IBS (IRRITABLE BOWEL SYNDROME)

Irritable bowel syndrome (IBS) is a common chronic gastrointestinal disorder. It is widely believed that IBS is caused by a deficient intake of dietary fiber, and most physicians recommend that patients with IBS increase their intake of dietary fiber in order to relieve their symptoms.

An attack of IBS can be triggered by emotional tension and anxiety, poor dietary habits and certain medications. Increased amounts of fiber in the diet can help relieve the symptoms of irritable bowel syndrome by producing soft, bulky stools. This helps to normalize the time it takes for the stool to pass through the colon. The effects of type of fiber have been documented in the management of IBS, and it is known to improve the overall symptoms in patients with IBS.

INFLAMMATORY BOWEL DISEASE

THE GASTROINTESTINAL SYSTEM

The GI tract consists of a series of mostly hollow organs beginning at the mouth, followed by the esophagus, stomach, small intestine, colon, rectum and anus. The roles of the gastrointestinal system are:

- Digestion
- Absorption of nutrients and water
- Elimination of waste

EFFECT

In people with Inflammatory Bowel Disease, inflammation in the organs of the digestive tract can affect the process of digestion. Inflammation in the small intestine of a person with Crohn's disease can interfere with the digestion and absorption of nutrients. Incompletely digested food that travels through the colon may cause diarrhea and abdominal pain. In a person with ulcerative colitis, the small intestine works normally, but the inflamed colon does not absorb water properly, resulting in diarrhea, increased urgency to have a bowel movement and increased frequency of bowel movements

FIBER & WEIGHT

If you suddenly start eating a lot of high-fiber foods, such as whole grains, fruits and veggies, you may get a little constipated from the large increase in fiber. Constipation is most likely if you don't drink plenty of water along with these fiber-filled foods. Gradually increase the amount of liquid you consume as you add more fiber to your diet to help limit the risk for constipation and other potential side effects, such as bloating and gas. Fiber is very filling, so the more you consume, the easier it is to decrease the total number of calories you're consuming and lose weight. It doesn't take much to get more fiber in your diet.

WATER & WEIGHT GAIN

Water and fiber don't cause permanent weight gain, in fact, they're often linked to weight loss. If you're experiencing unexplained weight gain, however, check with your doctor to make sure an underlying health issue isn't causing the problem.

If you drink two 8-ounce cups of water, then weigh yourself, your weight will go up about 1 pound, but it isn't caused by a gain of additional fat or muscle. As soon as the water works its way through your system, the extra pound will go away.

Eating a lot of carbohydrates, consuming a large amount of sodium and not drinking enough water during the day can cause your body to retain extra water, temporarily pushing your number on the scale upward.

FIBER & CROHNS DISEASE

Crohn's Disease is a chronic, recurrent inflammatory disease of the intestinal tract. There is now evidence of a genetic link as Crohn's frequently shows up in families and certain ethnic groups. A reduction in red meat is likely helpful. So is reducing the fat in the diet, including vegetable oils. More importantly, people who had low fiber ingestion in the diet had a greater chance of getting CD.

So, a gradual increase in the amount of fiber is likely helpful in hopefully preventing the disease. This should always be done in conjunction with the physician. It should be done gradually and should include soluble fibers which fertilize the best colon bacteria.

FIBER & DIARRHEA

When your stool is loose because there's too much water in your colon. Fiber can help get your system back in order in this case. Soluble fiber can actually absorb excess fluid in the bowel and thus act to firm up a loose stool. Insoluble fiber, which is not digestible, may help with constipation but make diarrhea worse

TOO MUCH FIBER INTAKE

A diet rich in fiber is essential for keeping the digestive system healthy. It is also related to lower blood pressure and a reduced risk of heart problems, diabetes, and obesity. When eating foods, such as high-fiber nutrition bars and fiber-added bread, eating 70 g of fiber in a day is not difficult.

Fiber makes bowel movements bigger and bulkier. It also promotes fermentation and gas formation. This is why excessive fiber intake frequently affects the digestive system.

Fiber is vital for healthy, solid bowel movements. However, too much of it can cause constipation. In this study, individuals who reduced their fiber intake had more frequent bowel movements, less bloating, and less abdominal pain that those who did not change their fiber intake.

TREATMENT

The symptoms of eating too much fiber can be reduced by:

- reducing fiber consumption
- increasing fluid consumption
- getting more exercise

- avoiding food that increases bloating, such as chewing gum

A person with severe symptoms may choose to adopt a low-fiber diet, which means eating 10 g of fiber a day until their symptoms can be better managed. This diet is most often prescribed for individuals with serious digestive conditions or after procedures.

SOURCES OF FIBER

There are two basic kinds of fiber, soluble and insoluble. Although the body cannot digest either of them, they are both necessary for a healthy diet.

Soluble fiber breaks down in the water found in the digestive system and forms a gel. It helps keep stools soft and slows the digestive process. Insoluble fiber does not break down at all, as it passes through the digestive system. It adds bulk to bowel movements and helps to move food along

It is essential to include a variety of fiber-rich foods in the diet. It's easy to add more fiber to your diet. Legumes are often the go-to source, because they're packed with fiber. A cup of canned low-sodium black beans has about 17 grams of fiber. A cup of cooked lentils has about 16 grams of fiber. A cup of canned low-sodium chickpeas (garbanzo beans) or pinto beans has about 11 grams of fiber.

FINAL WORD

Bottom line: You're likely not getting enough fiber, so consider eating more. The best way to get fiber is through natural sources, such as fruits, vegetables, whole grains, nuts, seeds, and legumes, because these sources also include important vitamins, minerals, and phytonutrients your body needs for optimal health.

GROCERY LIST WEEK 1

Unsweetened almond milk	Vanilla Protein powder	Cherry tomatoes	Strawberries	Whole-wheat bread	Mozzarella cheese	Kosher salt
Bananas	Honey	Bacon	Salt	Avocados	Tomatoes	Rice tortillas
Kale	Eggs	Butter	Pepper	Arugula leaves	Basil leaves	
Extra-virgin olive oil	Parsley	Boneless chicken breasts	Lemons	Mozzarella cheese	Tomatoes	Basil leaves
Cucumbers	Mayonnaise	Balsamic vinegar	Parmesan	½ pound whole wheat penne pasta	Red bell peppers	Yellow bell peppers
Capers	Oregano	Kalamata olives	Feta cheese	Broccoli	Zucchini	Cayenne pepper
Soy sauce	Brown rice	2 salmon fillets	2 steak	Mushrooms	Cherry tomatoes	Peanut butter
White veingar	Fish sauce	Stevia	Chicken	Celery	Carrots	Bay leaves
Nuts	Flax crackers	Chia seeds	Clementine	Walnuts		

MEAL PLAN WEEK 1

DAY	BREAKFAST	LUNCH	DINNER	SNACKS
MONDAY	Green smoothie	Chicken caprese wraps	Fried salmon	1 clementine 8 dried walnut halves
TUESDAY	Avocado caprese toast	Arugula salad	Avocado shrimp salad	Nuts Slices of cheese and bell peppers
WEDNESDAY	Green smoothie	Chicken caprese wraps	Fried salmon	Sticks of celery and pepper with guacamole
THURSDAY	Avocado caprese toast	Arugula salad	Avocado shrimp salad	Sticks of celery and pepper with guacamole
FRIDAY	Strawberry smoothie	Pasta salad	Beef salad	Nuts Slices of cheese and bell peppers
SATURDAY	Bacon & eggs	Brown rice with cooked veggies	Chicken soup	A boiled egg Flax crackers with cheese
SUNDAY	Strawberry smoothie	Pasta salad	Beef salad	Smoothie with almond milk, nut butter, chia seeds, and spinach

RECIPES WEEK 1

GREEN SMOOTHIE

NUTRITION :

343 calories; 14.2 g total fat, 54.7 g carbohydrates, 5.9 g protein

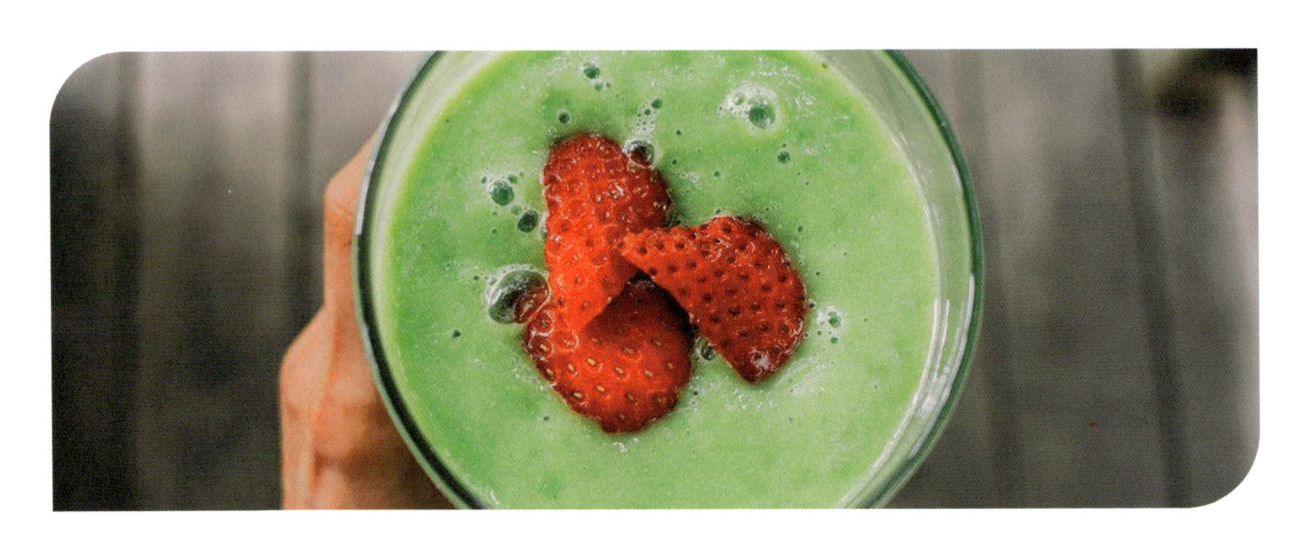

Ingredients

1 large ripe banana

1 cup kale

1 cup unsweetened vanilla almond milk

1 tbsp. Vanilla protein powder

2 teaspoons honey

1 cup ice cubes

RECIPE:

1. Put ingredients into the blender in the order listed.
2. Start blending on low speed and increase to high.
3. Blend on high speed for 50-60 seconds until mixture is smooth

BACON & EGGS

NUTRITION :

Calories 272kcal, Fat 22g, Carbs 1g, Protein 15g

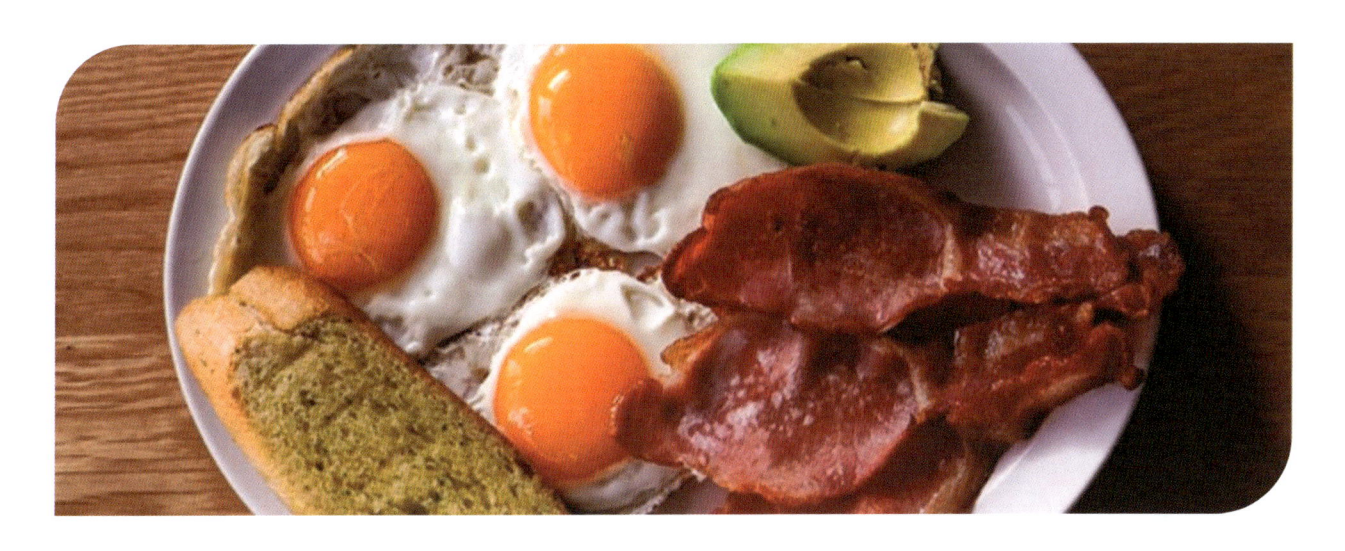

Ingredients

2 Eggs
1 ¼ oz bacon, slices
Cherry tomatoes
Butter
Salt & pepper

RECIPE:

1. Preheat your oven to 350 F
2. Lay the bacon on a cookie sheet and place into oven once it's heated.
3. Wait 10-15 minutes until crispy, and remove.
4. Use pan to fry the eggs. Place it over medium heat and crack your eggs into the bacon grease.
5. Cook the eggs any way you like them.
6. Salt and pepper to taste.

STRAWBERRY SMOOTHIE

NUTRITION :

Calories 152, fat 13g, carbs 5g, protein 1g, net carbs 4g

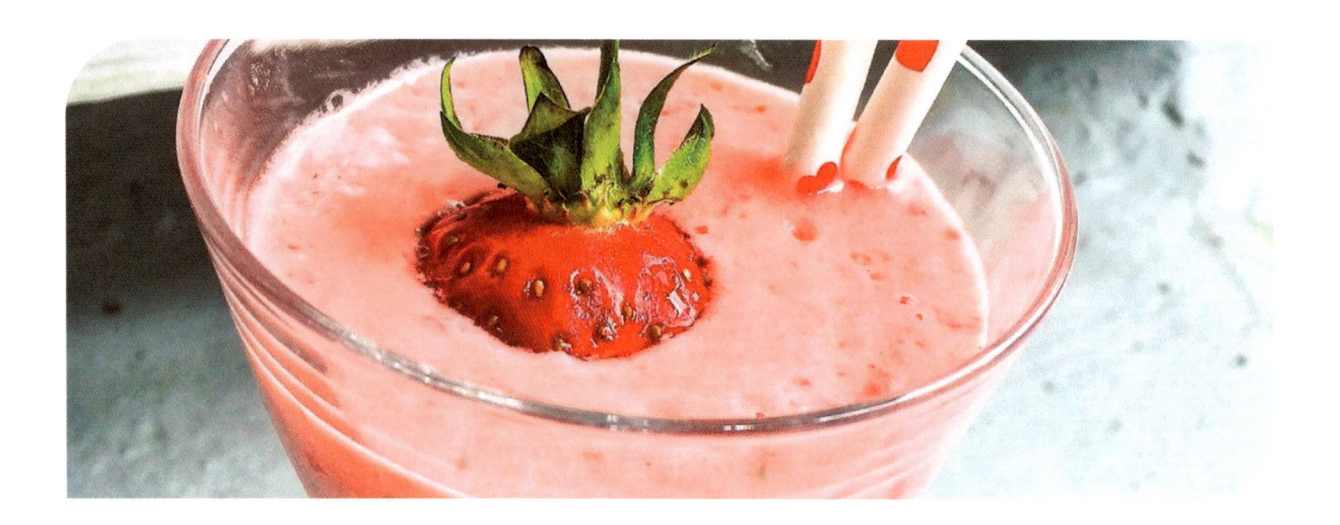

Ingredients

1 cup strawberries

Ice

2 cups Unsweetened almond milk

Whipping cream

½ tbsp. vanilla extract

RECIPE:

Put all the ingredients in a blender and blend until smooth.

Top with sliced strawberries and enjoy.

AVOCADO CAPRESE TOAST

NUTRITION :

Calories 173, Fat 11g, Carbs 16g, Protein 4g

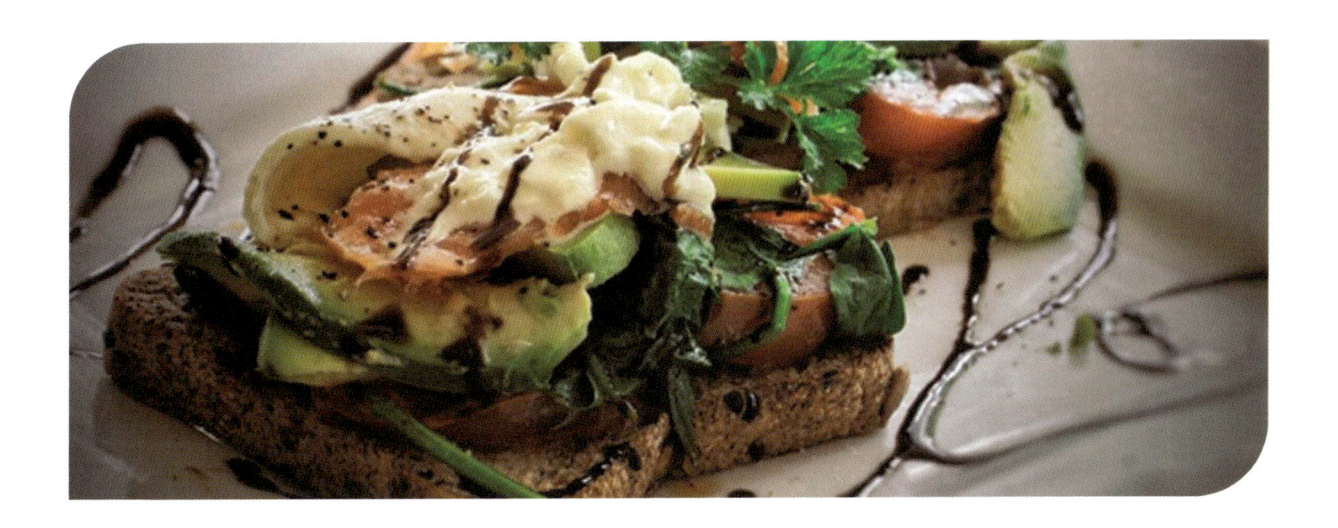

Ingredients

2 slice whole wheat bread

1/2 cup or so of fresh arugula leaves

1 ball fresh mozzarella cheese sliced

1 tomato sliced

1 avocado pitted and sliced

basil leaves

kosher salt and freshly ground black pepper

RECIPE:

Layer slices of tomato, mozzarella cheese and avocado on a toast. Add a few torn pieces of basil leaves. Season with kosher salt and pepper.

CHICKEN CAPRESE WRAPS

NUTRITION :

Calories 612, Fat 32g, Carbs 46g, Protein 34g

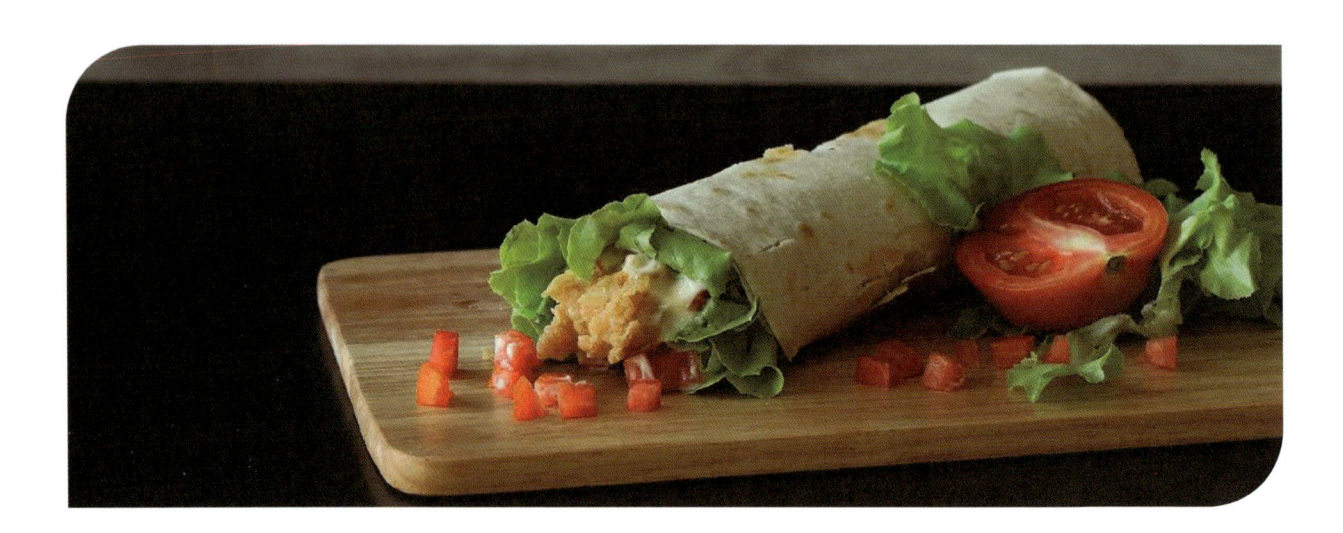

Ingredients

3 tablespoons extra virgin olive oil divided, plus more for drizzling

1 teaspoon fresh parsley minced

½ lemon juiced

kosher salt and freshly ground black pepper

2 skinless boneless chicken breasts

Rice Tortillas

1 8 ounce mozzarella cheese sliced

3-4 medium tomatoes, chopped

¼ cup fresh basil leaves

balsamic vinegar

mayonnaise

cucumbers

RECIPE:

1. Mix 2 tablespoons of extra virgin olive oil, parsley, lemon juice and salt and pepper in a medium size bowl. Add the chicken breasts and turn to coat and let the chicken stand at room temperature.
2. Light a grill and set to high or prepare a grill pan on the stove and heat to medium high heat. Discard the marinade and add the chicken to the grill or pan and season with more salt and pepper. After about 3-4 minutes, turn the chicken breasts. Cook for another 3 minutes. If on the grill, turn off one side of the grill and move chicken to that side, cover and cook until chicken has an internal temperature of 185 degrees. If on the stove, reduce the heat to medium, cover and cook until chicken has an internal temperature of 185 degrees. Slice the chicken and set aside.
3. Layer all the ingredients in tortillas and fold the tortillas.

ARUGULA SALAD

NUTRITION :

Calories 40, Fat 3g, Carbs 2.5g, Protein 0.5g

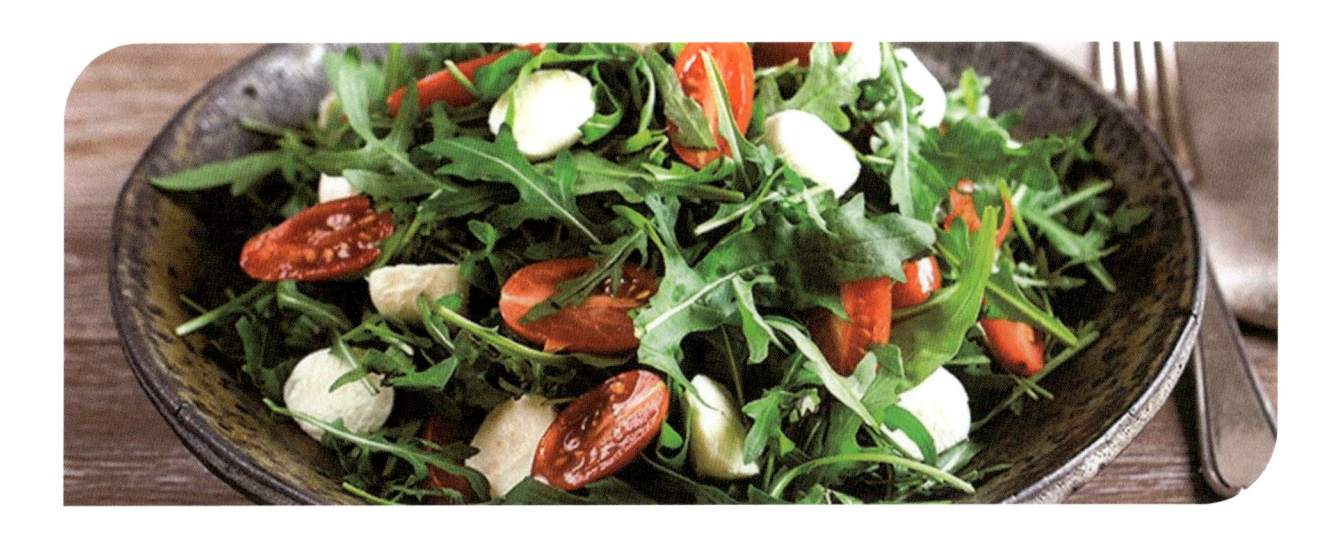

Ingredients

2 bunch arugula
6 tbsp. extra-virgin olive oil
2 tbsp. lemon juice
Kosher salt
Freshly ground black pepper
Parmesan

RECIPE:

Make dressing: In a medium bowl, whisk together olive oil and lemon juice, then season with salt and pepper.

In a large bowl, lightly dress arugula, then top with Parmesan.

PASTA SALAD

NUTRITION :

400 calories; 24.8 g fat; 39 g carbohydrates; 7.9 g protein

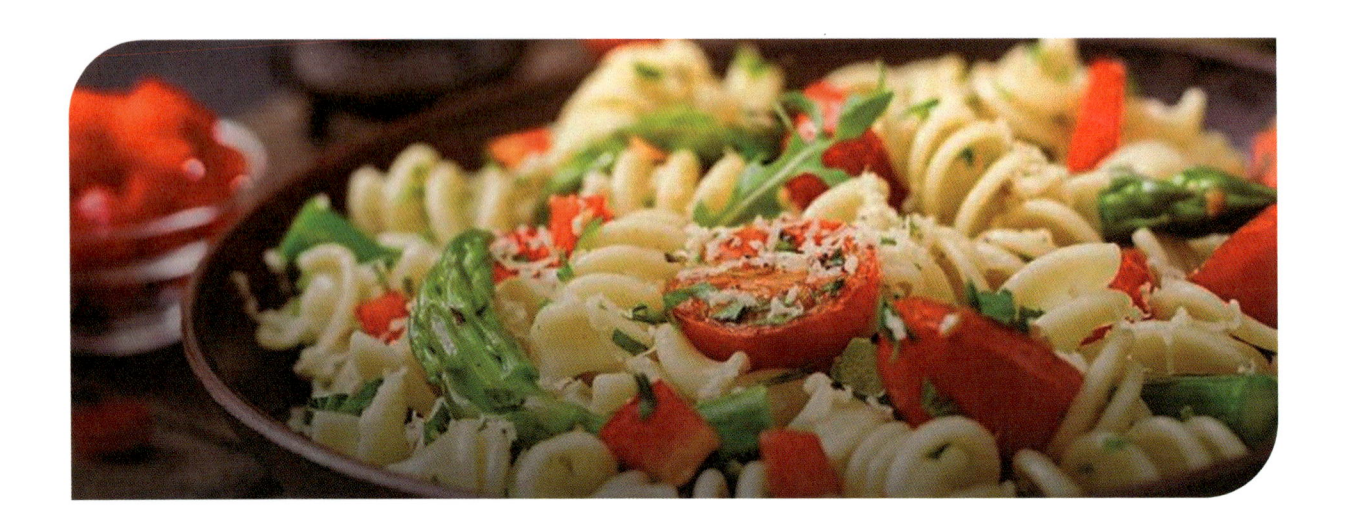

Ingredients

1/2 pound whole wheat penne pasta

2 medium tomatoes chopped

1/3 cup roasted red and/or yellow bell pepper roughly chopped

2 tablespoons capers drained

1/4 cup sliced kalamata olives sliced in half

1/4 cup extra virgin olive oil

1 tablespoon balsamic vinegar

2 cloves of garlic minced or pressed

1/2 teaspoon oregano

pinch of sugar

kosher salt and freshly ground black pepper

1/2 cup basil slivered

1/4 cup feta cheese

RECIPE:

1. In a large pot of salted boiling water, cook pasta until al dente, rinse under cold water and drain.
2. Whisk together the salad spice mix and Italian dressing.
3. In a salad bowl, combine the pasta, cherry tomatoes, bell peppers and olives. Pour dressing over salad; toss and refrigerate overnight.

BROWN RICE WITH VEGETABLES

NUTRITION :

Calories: 197 Sugar: 3.5g
Sodium: 476.8 mg Fat: 7.9 g,
Protein: 5.6g

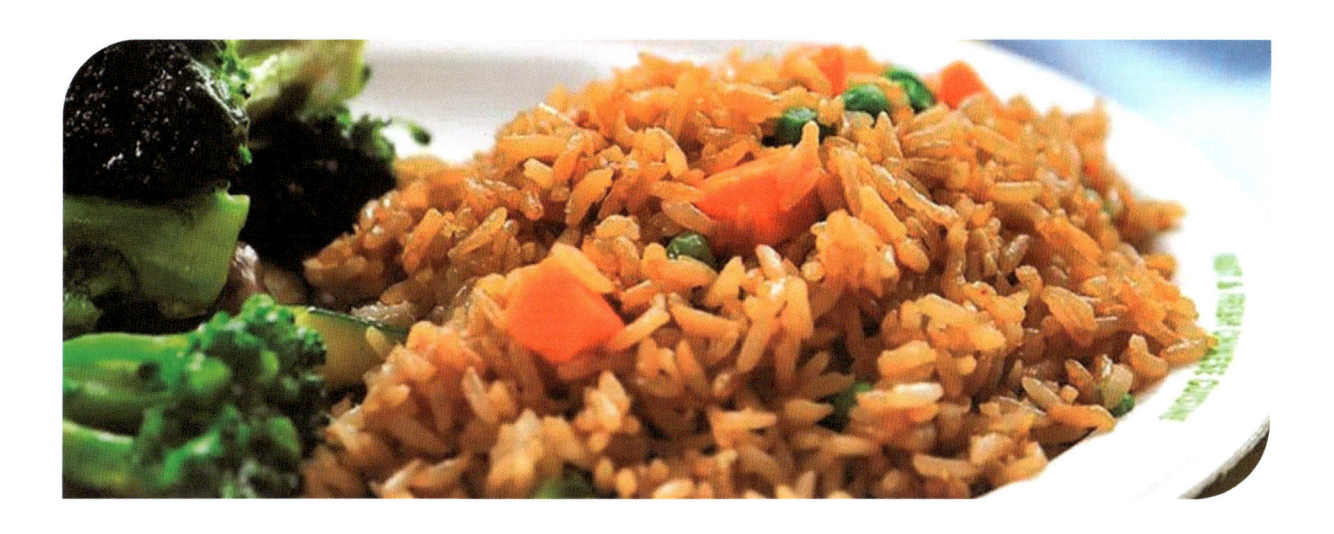

Ingredients

1/2 head of broccoli, chopped

1/2 chopped red bell pepper

1/2 chopped zucchini

2 tbsp extra virgin olive oil

4 cloves of garlic, minced

1 handful fresh parsley, finely chopped

1/8 tsp cayenne powder

2 tbsp tamari or soy sauce

1 cup brown rice

6 cups water

Salt

RECIPE:

1. Add 6 cups of water and a pinch of salt into a large pot and place it over the heat to boil. Rinse the rice under running water
2. Add the rice into the boiling water
3. Adjust the temperature reduce accordingly.
4. Boil it for at least 25-30 minutes or until soft uncovered .
5. drain the water from the rice and shift the rice back to the pot and let it rest for 5-10 minutes.
6. Add some water in a pan and bring it to a boil. Then add the veggies and cook for 1 to 2 minutes over high-heat. Drain the veggies and set aside.
7. Heat the oil in the wok and add the garlic, cayenne powder and parsley. Cook over high-heat for about 1 minute, stirring occasionally.
8. Add the vegetables, rice and tamari. Cook for about 1 to 2 minutes more.

FRIED SALMON

NUTRITION :

Calories 525kcal, Fat 24g, Carbs 0.3g, Protein 31g

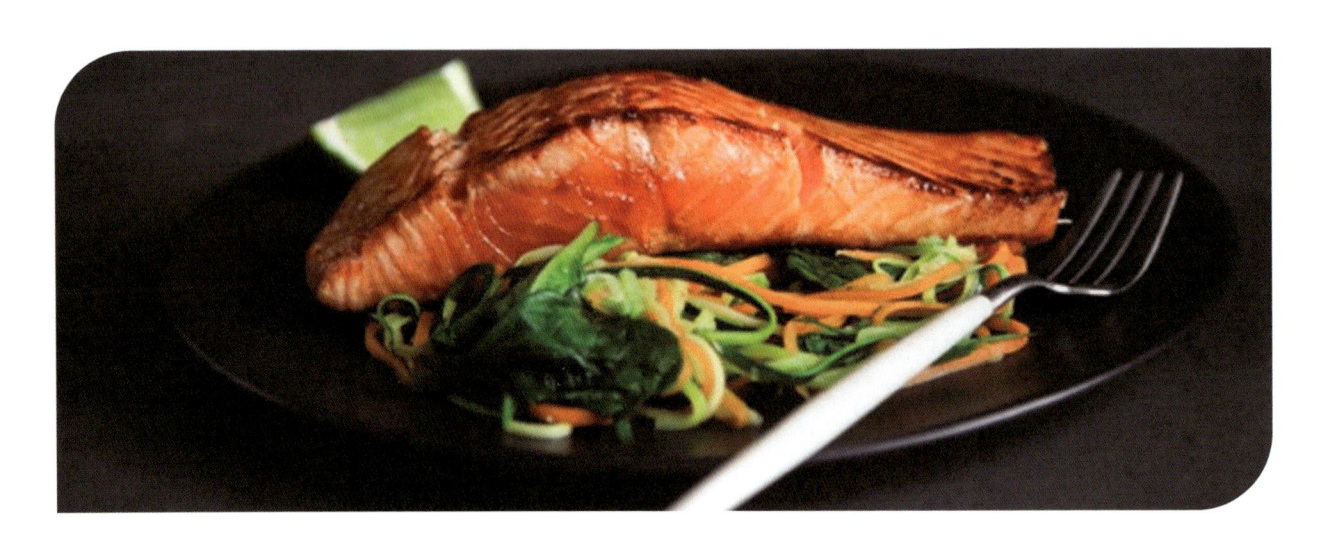

Ingredients

2 salmon fillets
1 or 2 tbsp olive oil
1 lemon
Salt
Pepper

RECIPE:

1. Put a non-stick frying pan on medium heat and add olive oil.
2. Season the salmon with salt and pepper.
3. Add the salmon fillets in the pan and fry until its crispy or golden.
4. Top with lemon juice.

BEEF SALAD

NUTRITION :

Calories 784kcal, Fat 66g, Carbs 3g, Protein 43g

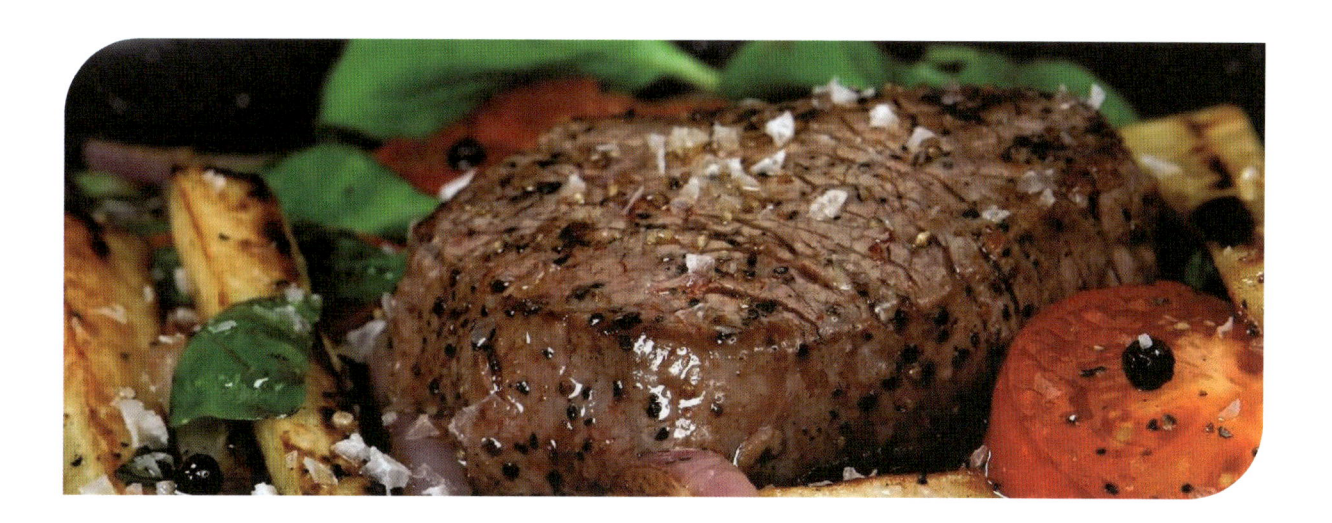

Ingredients

300g steak
Mushrooms
2 tbsp olive oil
1 garlic clove, minced
Sea salt
Pepper
Cherry tomatoes, halved
Mixed greens
11 oz. drained baby mozzarella

Dressing

olive oil
1 Tbsp Peanut Butter
1 Clove garlic, minced
1 Tsp Soya Sauce
1 Tsp White Vinegar
1 Squirt Fish Sauce
1 Squeeze Lime juice
2 Drops Stevia
Salt & Pepper to taste

RECIPE:

1. Pre-heat a pan on the stovetop, or outdoor grill over medium-high heat.
2. Season the steak with salt and pepper. Combine the olive oil and garlic in a small bowl and then brush it over all sides of the steak.
3. Sear the steak for 3-4 minutes per side, depending upon the thickness of the fillet, for medium-rare steaks.
4. Remove from the heat and cover loosely with foil. Rest for 5 minutes.
5. For the dressing mix all the ingredients in a bowl and whisk together to emulsify and form the dressing

CHICKEN SOUP

NUTRITION :

Calories 157, Fat 3g, Carbs 19g, Protein 15g

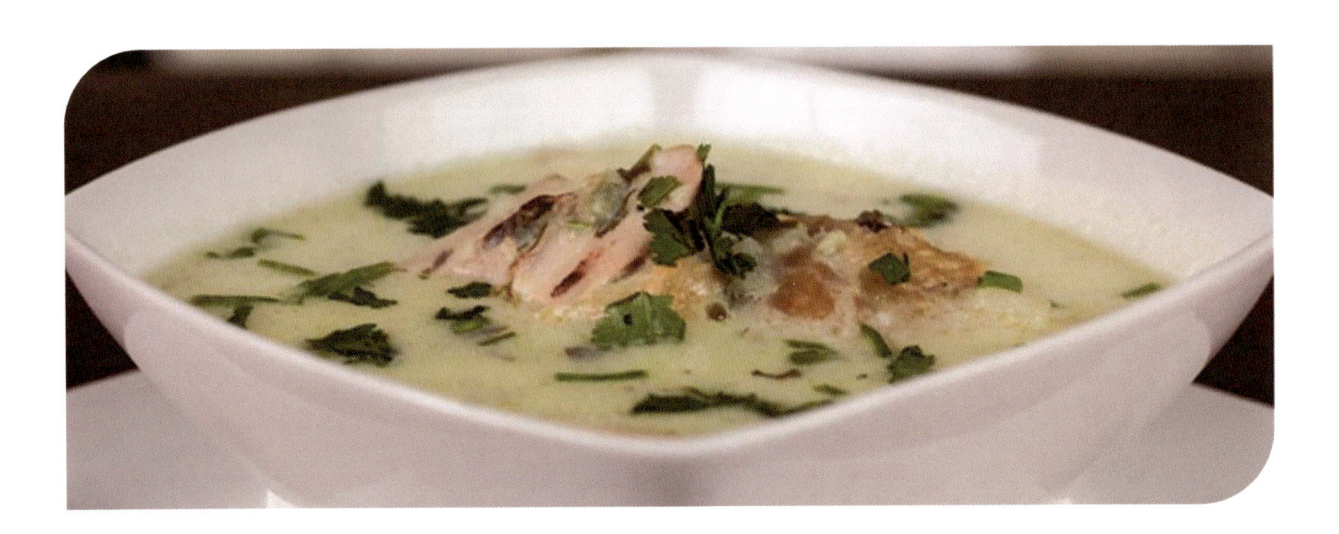

Ingredients

1 (3 pound) whole chicken

4 cups low-sodium chicken broth

2 carrots, sliced

2 celery stalks, sliced

1 medium onion, chopped

1 bay leaf

2 tablespoons chopped parsley

RECIPE:

1. Put the chicken, carrots, celery and onion in a large soup pot and cover with cold water. Heat and simmer, uncovered, until the chicken is soft and boiled.
2. Take everything out. set aside to cool. Add the carrots, celery, onion and bay leaf to the broth, bring back to a simmer and cook until the vegetables are about half cooked (they will still have resistance when tested with a knife but be somewhat pliable when bent), about 10 minutes.
3. Return the chicken and everything to the pot, stir and serve.

GROCERY LIST WEEK 2

Butter	*Blueberries*	*Vanilla extract*	*Baking powder*	*Baby spinach*	*Red onions extra-virgin olive oil*	*Red vinegar*
Eggs	*Whipping cream*	*Bacon*	*Olive oil*	*English cucumbers*	*2 15oz can hearts of palm*	*Vegetable oil*
Salt	*Coconut powder*	*Cherry tomatoes*	*Avocados*	*Carrots*	*Italian parsley*	*Kosher salt*
Pepper	*Milk/ unsweetened almond milk*	*Bananas*	*Zucchini*	*2 15oz can tuna in oil*	*Red onions*	*Quinoa*
Red bell pepper	*Yellow bell pepper*	*Balsamic vinegar*	*Vegetable stock*	*300g steak*	*Garlic*	*Mushrooms*
11oz baby mozzarella	*½ pound whole wheat penne pasta*	*kalamata olives*	*Capers*	*Oregano*	*Basil*	*Feta cheese*
All-purpose flour	*Mozzarella cheese*	*Cream cheese*	*Unsweetened tomato sauce*	*Pepperoni*	*Almond flour*	*Italian seasoning*

MEAL PLAN WEEK 2

DAY	BREAKFAST	LUNCH	DINNER	SNACKS
MONDAY	Blueberry smoothie	Avocado egg salad	Quinoa bowl	Bowl of mixed berries
TUESDAY	Scrambled eggs	Chicken gyros	Vegetable & bean salad	A handful of nuts
WEDNESDAY	Banana Pancakes	Avocado egg salad	Beef salad	Bowl of sliced cucumbers
THURSDAY	Blueberry smoothie	Pasta salad	Quinoa bowl	Hard-boiled egg with salt
FRIDAY	Scrambled eggs	Avocado tuna salad	Tomato & hearts of palm salad	Fruit salad
SATURDAY	Banana Pancakes	Chicken gyros	Vegetable & bean salad	2 bananas
SUNDAY	Eggs & bacon	Avocado tuna salad	Tomato & hearts of palm salad	1 bowl of cherry tomatoes/ 1 orange

BLUEBERRY SMOOTHIE

NUTRITION :

211 calories; 3.9 g fat; 35.5 g carbohydrates; 9.5 g protein

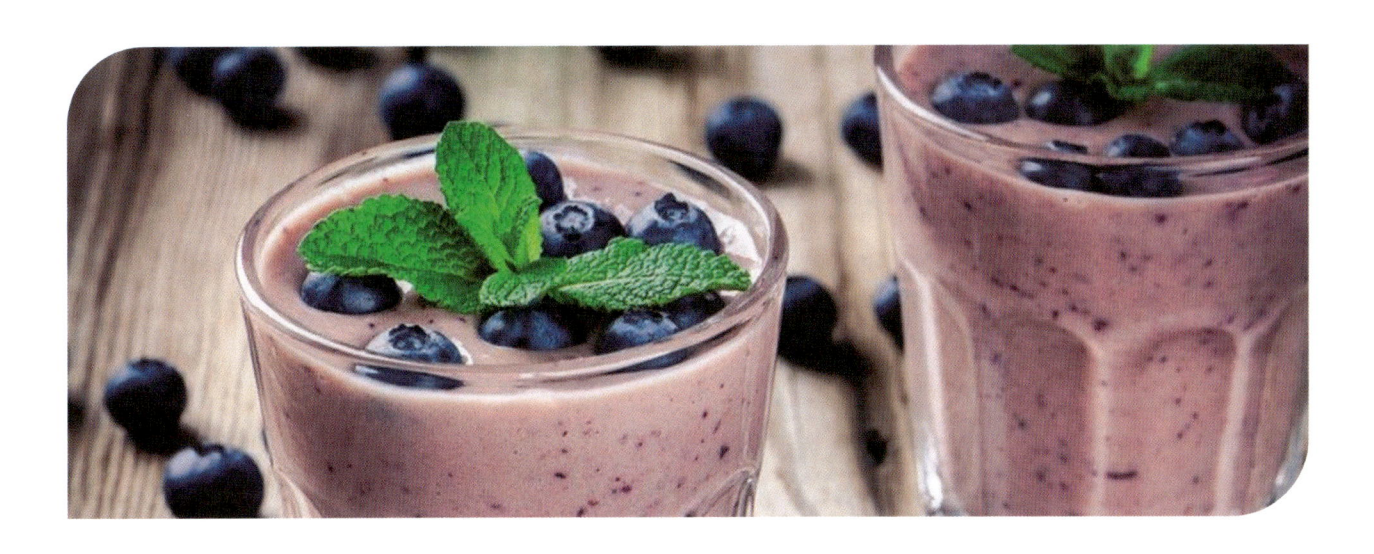

Ingredients

2 cup unsweetened almond milk

½ tbsp. vanilla extract

Whipping cream

Ice

Blueberries 1 cup

RECIPE:

Mix together all the ingredients in a blender and blend until smooth.

Pour the smoothie in a glass and enjoy.

SCRAMBLED EGGS

NUTRITION :

Calories 327kcal, Fat 31g, Carbs 1g, Protein 11g

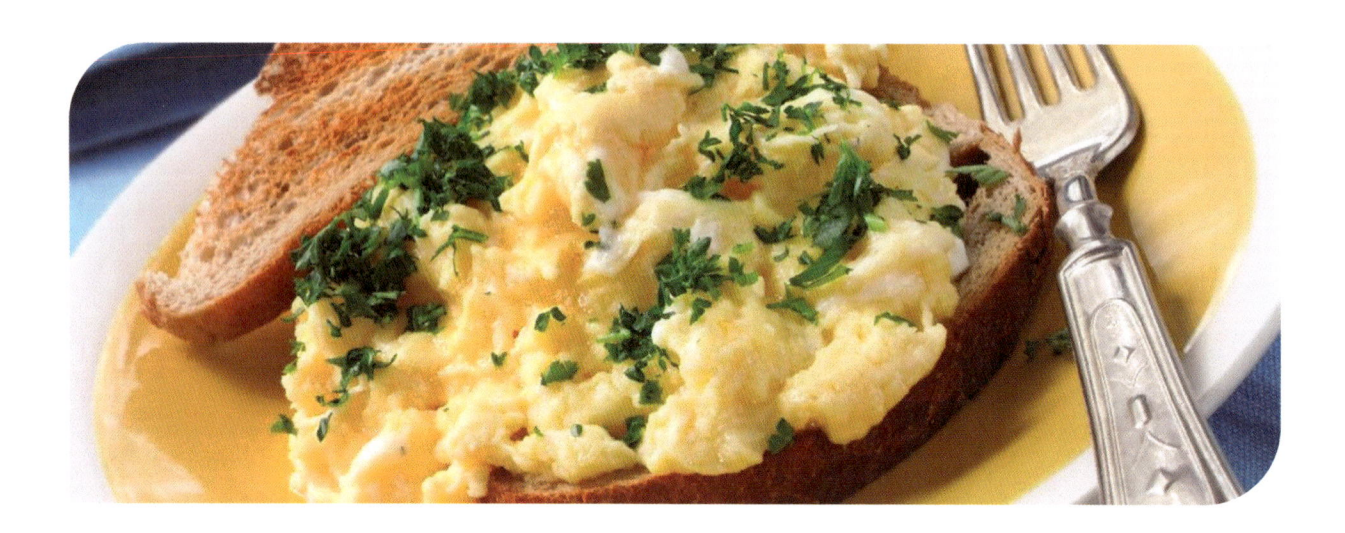

Ingredients

1 oz. butter
2 eggs
salt and pepper

RECIPE:

1. Crack the eggs into a small bowl and use a fork to whisk them together with some salt and pepper.
2. Heat butter in large nonstick skillet over medium heat until hot. POUR in egg mixture. As eggs begin to set, gently PULL the eggs across the pan with a spatula, forming large soft curds.
3. Continue cooking—pulling, lifting and folding eggs—until thickened and no visible liquid egg remains. Remember that the eggs will still be cooking even after you've put them on your plate.

BANANA PANCAKES

NUTRITION :

Calories 248, Fat 10g, Carbs 25g, Protein 13g

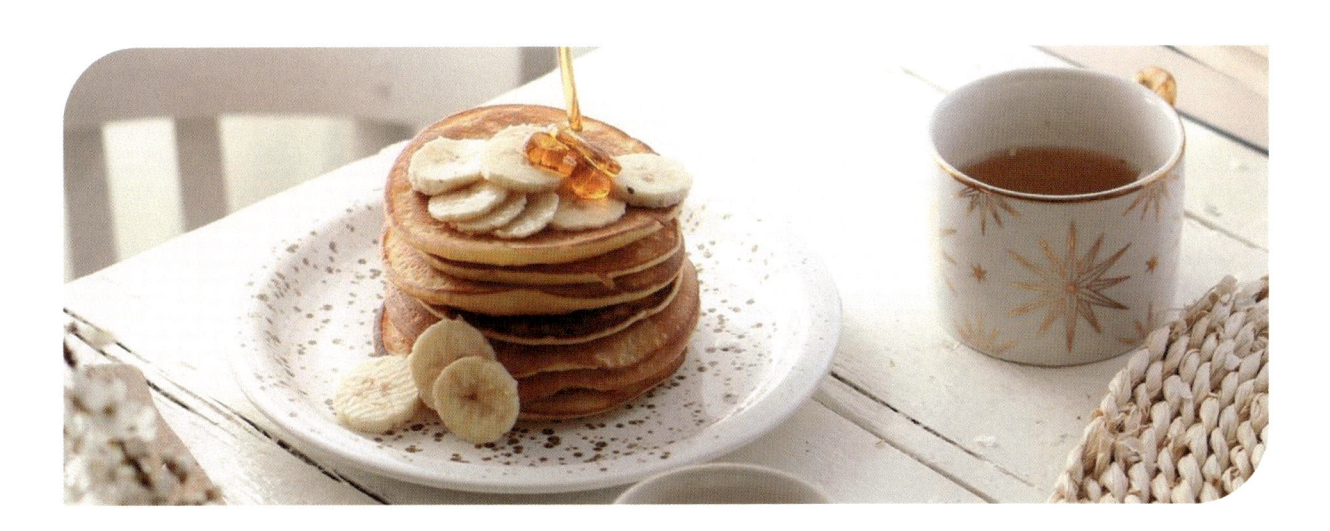

Ingredients

1 banana
2 eggs, beaten
Baking powder
Vanilla extract
½ tbsp oil
All-purpose flour 1 cup

RECIPE:

1. In a medium bowl, mash 1 large banana with a fork until it is mashed completely.
2. Mixing in 2 beaten eggs, a touch of baking powder and a squish of vanilla extract.
3. Heat a large non-stick frying pan over a medium heat and brush with ½ tbsp oil.
4. Using half of the mixture, spoon two pancakes into the pan.
5. Cook each side for about 2 minutes and remove from heat and put it on a plate.

AVOCADO EGG SALAD

NUTRITION :

Calories: 213, Total fat: 16 g, Carbohydrates: 9 g, Protein: 9 g

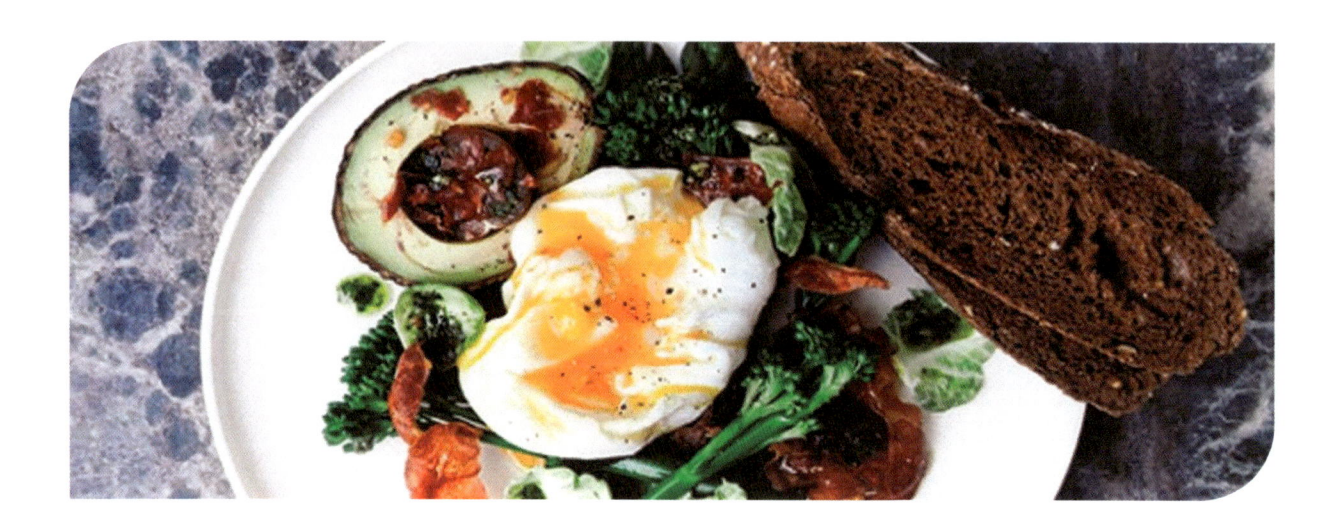

Ingredients

½ medium avocado, sliced

1 hard-boiled egg, cut into slices

2 Cherry tomatoes, halved

Baby spinach

Zucchini noodles

Chia seeds

English cucumber

1 medium carrot, chopped

Salt and pepper

RECIPE:

Add all the ingredients in a bowl and season with salt and pepper. Add chia seeds on top.

AVOCADO TUNA SALAD

NUTRITION :

Calories 304, Fats 20g, Carbs 9g, Protein 22g

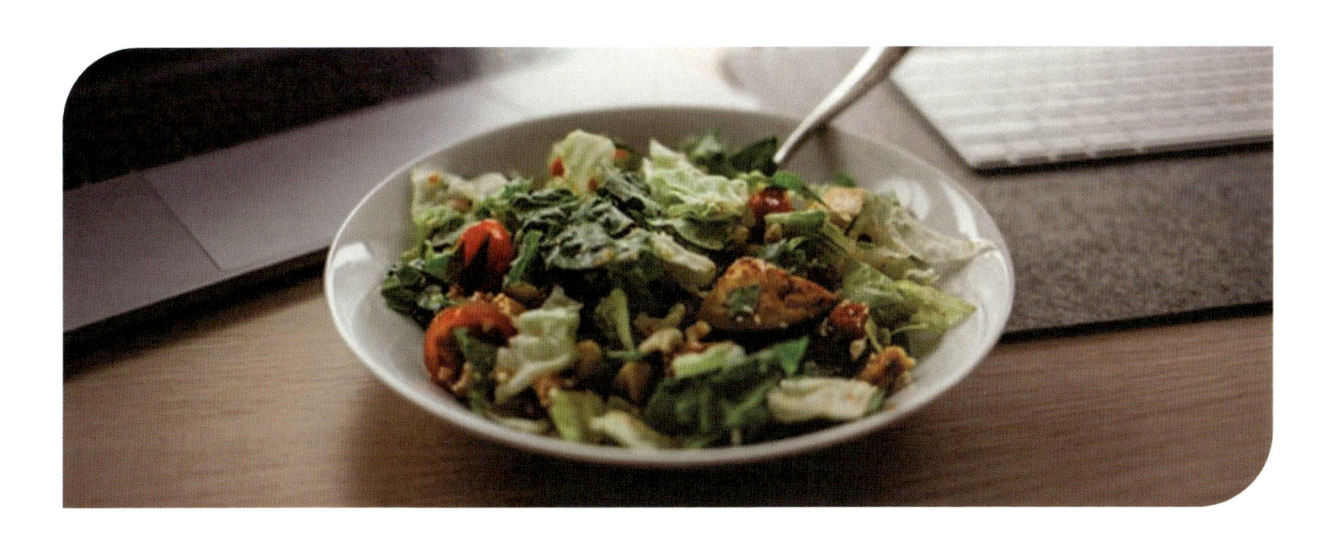

Ingredients

15 oz tuna in oil, drained

1 English cucumber, sliced

1 medium avocado, chopped

1 small/medium red onion, sliced

Salt

Freshly ground black pepper

Extra-virgin olive oil

Lemon juice

Lemon zest

RECIPE:

Mix all the ingredients in a bowl and season with salt, olive oil, lemon juice and pepper.

TOMATO & HEARTS OF PALM SALAD

NUTRITION :

Calories: 90.6kcal, Carbohydrates: 9g, Protein: 2.3g, Fat: 6.3g

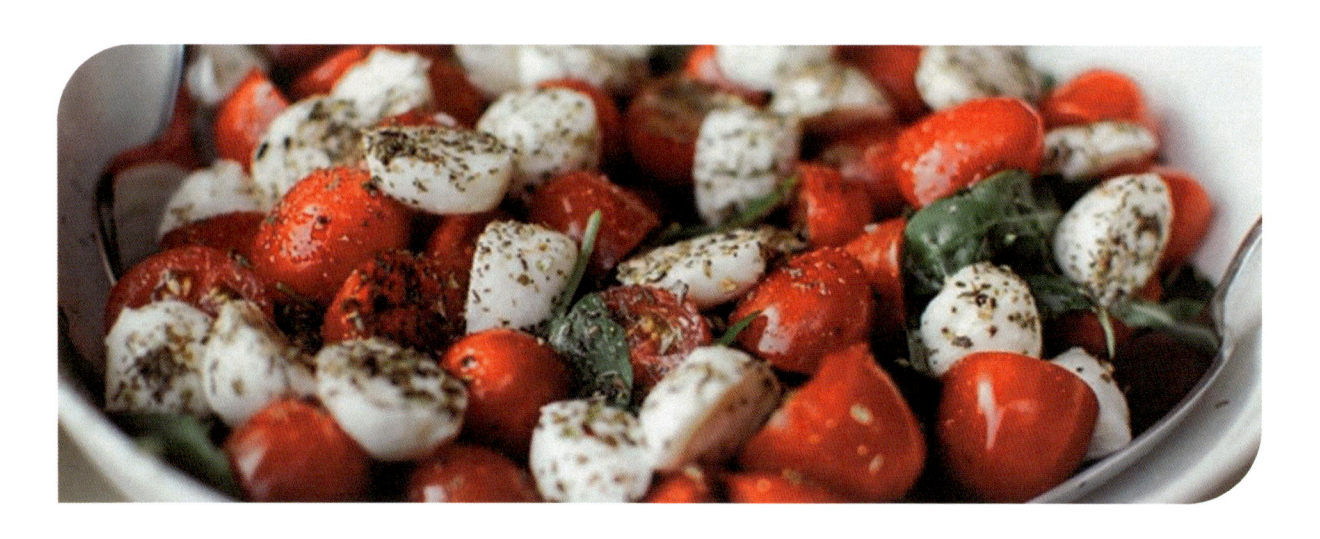

Ingredients

3 cups cherry tomatoes sliced in half

1 15- ounce can hearts of palm drained and sliced into 1/4 inch rings

1/4 cup thinly sliced or shaved red onion

1/4 cup chopped Italian parsley

1/4 cup vegetable oil

1 1/2 tablespoon red vinegar

1 teaspoon sugar

1 teaspoon kosher salt

1/2 teaspoon freshly ground black pepper

RECIPE:

Combine tomatoes, hearts of palm, red onion and all the ingredients in a small bowl and mix. Add salt and pepper to taste.

QUINOA BOWL

NUTRITION :

Calories: 341kcal,
Carbohydrates: 7g,
Protein: 28g, Fat: 21g

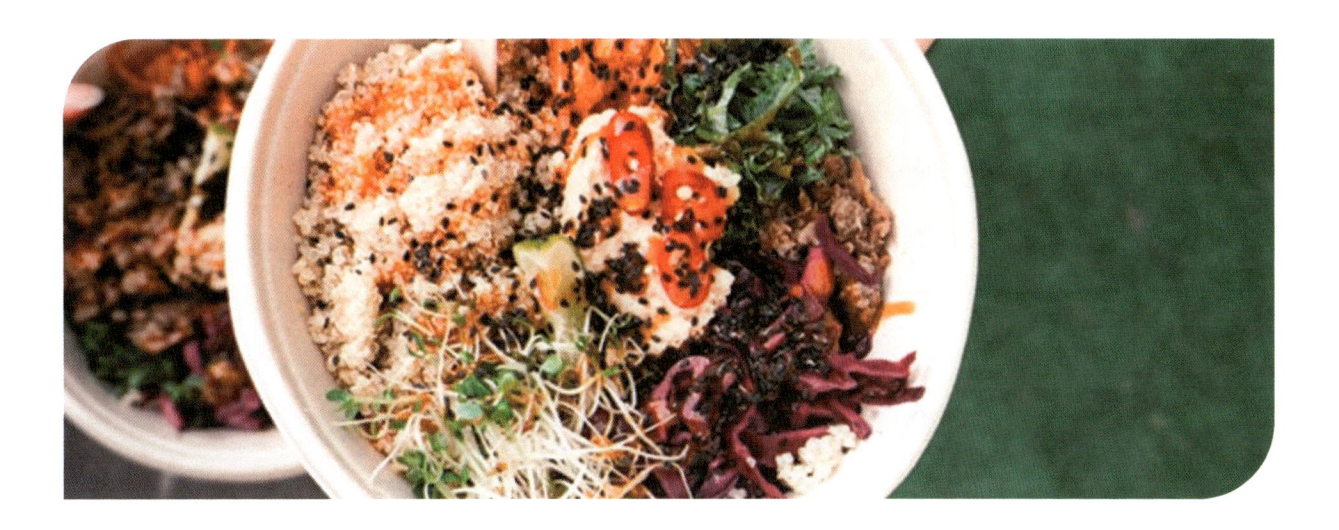

Ingredients

1 cup quinoa, rinsed
2 cups vegetable stock
Cherry tomatoes
Salt
Pepper
Lemon juice
Red onions
Red bell pepper
Yellow bell pepper
Cucumber, sliced
Balsamic vinegar
Baby spinach

RECIPE:

1. Pour rinsed quinoa and vegetable stock in a medium saucepan and cover with a lid. Bring to a boil. Once the quinoa has begun to boil, reduce to a simmer, cover and cook for 15-20 minutes. Remove from heat and set aside.
2. Assemble all the ingredients in a bowl and add quinoa in the bowl.
3. Sprinkle some salt and pepper on top.

GROCERY LIST WEEK 3

Bananas + All-purpose flour	Balsamic vinegar	Unsweetened Almond milk	Avocados	Carrots	Hummus
Vanilla extract	Mozzarella	Apples	Oranges	Grapes	Salad greens
Eggs	Cucumbers	Kiwis	Mangoes	Honey	Radish
Berries	Tomatoes	Strawberries	Blueberries	Raspberries	1 oz dark chocolate
Plain Greek nonfat yogurt	Boneless chicken breasts	Celery	Pecans	Red onions	Nuts
Yellow onions	Olive oil	Garlic	2 14oz can low-sodium chicken broth	2 (14.5 oz) cans diced tomatoes	Potatoes
Parsley	Bay leaves	Thyme	Corn	Peas	½ pound whole wheat penne pasta
Tomatoes	Kalamata olives	Yellow bell pepper	Red bell pepper	Capers	Balsamic vinegar
Oregano	Feta cheese	Basil leaves	Red onions	Sweet onions	Cilantro
Green bell pepper	Vegetable broth	Portobello mushroom	Asparagus	Dill	Mint
Kale	Chicken fillets	2 7oz bag baby spinach	Grape tomatoes	Sweet	Baking powder

MEAL PLAN WEEK 3

DAY	BREAKFAST	LUNCH	DINNER	SNACKS
MONDAY	Avocado banana smoothie	Veggie & hummus salad	Avocado salad	Sliced tomato, mozzarella and balsamic vinegar
TUESDAY	Avocado banana smoothie	Avocado & chicken salad	Chopped grilled vegetable salad	1 large banana and carrot sticks
WEDNESDAY	Oats with fruits & seeds toppings	Veggie soup	Chopped grilled vegetable salad	1 cup sliced cucumbers
THURSDAY	Oats with fruits & seeds topping	Veggie soup	Bowl of kale with strawberries & avocado	1 oz dark chocolate
FRIDAY	Fruit salad	Veggie & hummus salad	Chicken spinach salad	1 apple and a handful of nuts
SATURDAY	Fruit salad	Avocado & chicken salad	Bowl of kale with strawberries & avocado	1 hard-boiled egg
SUNDAY	Pancakes	Pasta salad	Chicken spinach salad	Cup of berries

AVOCADO BANANA SMOOTHIE

NUTRITION :

Calories 146, Fat 6g, Carbs 16g, Protein 6g

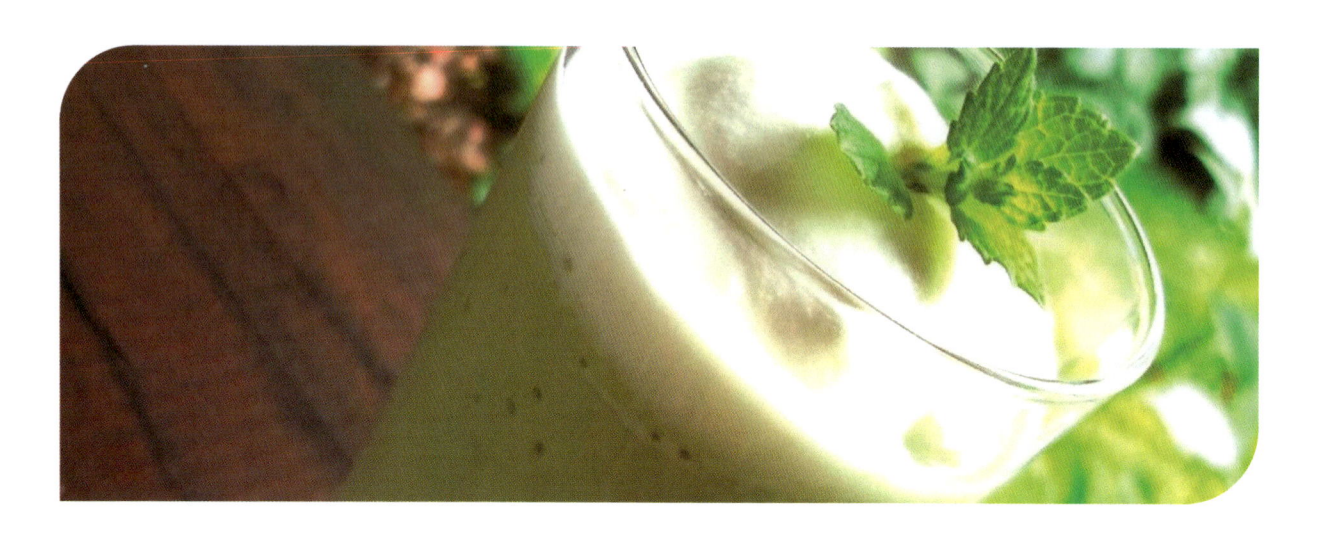

Ingredients

1 large banana
½ medium avocado
1 tsp. vanilla extract
1 cup unsweetened almond milk

RECIPE:

Add banana, avocado, almond milk and vanilla extract to the high speed blender and blend until smooth.

FRUIT SALAD

NUTRITION :

155 calories; 0.6 g fat; 39 g carbohydrates; 1.8 g protein

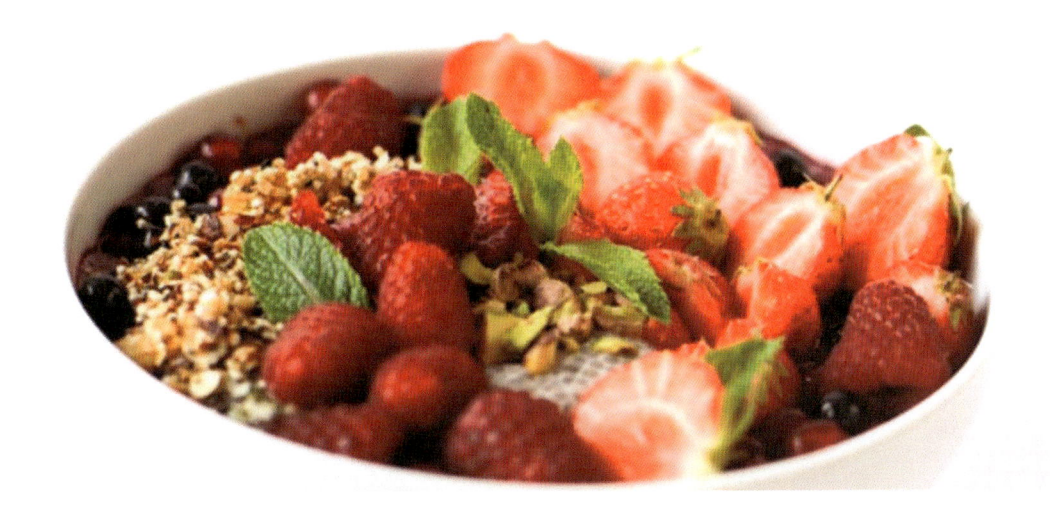

Ingredients

½ cup strawberries, hulled and quarter

½ cup blueberries

½ cup raspberries

3 kiwis, peeled and sliced

1 orange, peeled and wedges cut in half

2 apples, peeled and chopped

1 mango, peeled and chopped

2 c. grapes

1/4 c. honey

Zest of 1 lemon

RECIPE:

In a small bowl whisk together honey, orange juice, and lemon zest. Add fruit to a large bowl and pour over dressing, tossing gently to combine.

VEGETABLE & HUMMUS SALAD

NUTRITION :

Calories 543kcal, Fat 28g, Protein 10g, Carbs 66.4g

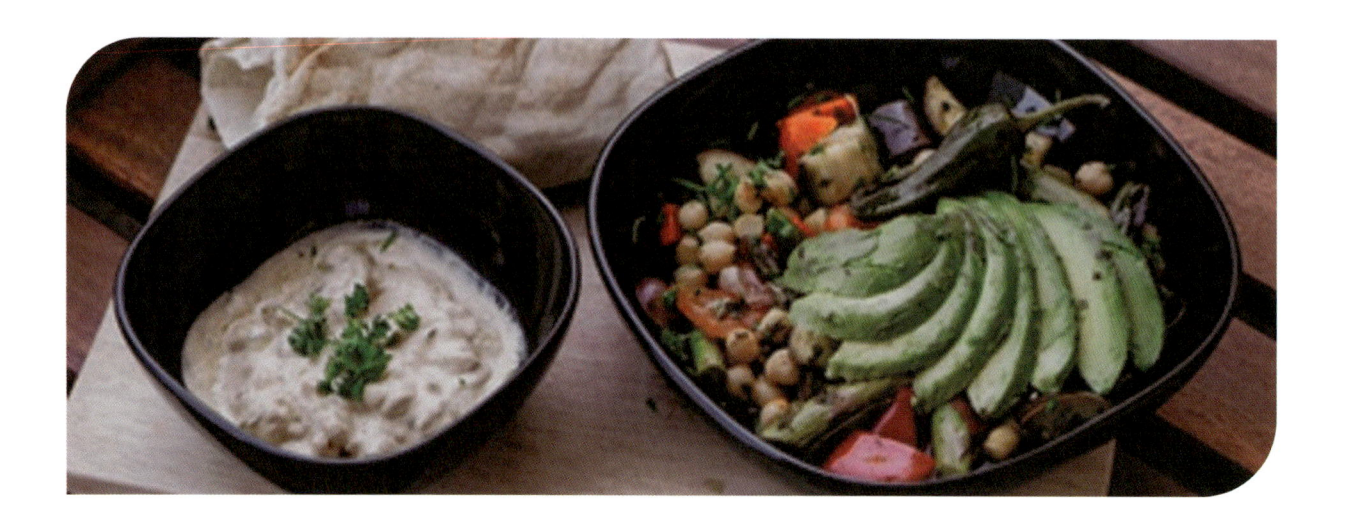

Ingredients

1 Medium onion
Lemon juice
1 cucumber
Salad greens
Carrots
Radish
Any other veggies of your choice

RECIPE:

Put the onions, carrots, cucumber and the other veggies into a bowl .

Top with a spoon or two of hummus and put some lemon juice on top.

AVOCADO & CHICKEN SALAD

NUTRITION :

Calories 359, Fat 19g, Carbs 23g, Protein 27g

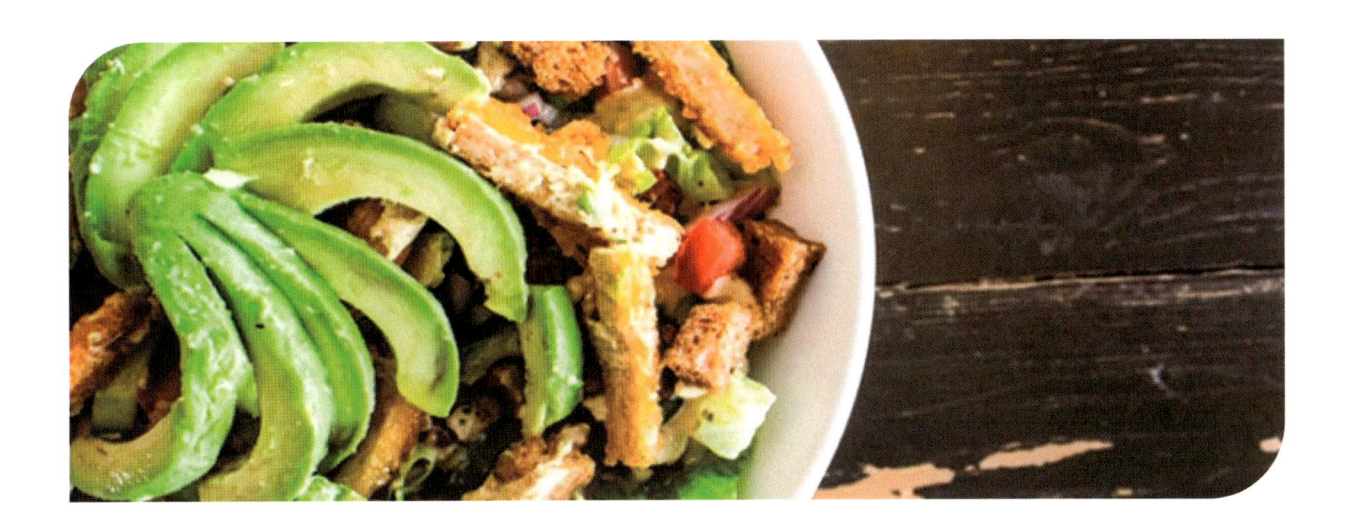

Ingredients

1 cup plain Greek Nonfat Yogurt

1 avocado , mashed

1-2 tablespoons fresh lemon juice

Kosher salt and freshly ground black pepper

2 cups shredded chicken (from about 16 ounces of skinless, boneless breast)

3/4 cup chopped celery (about 2 ribs)

1/2 cup red grapes , halved

1/3 cup chopped pecans

1/3 cup chopped red onion

RECIPE:

In a small bowl, mix the nonfat Greek yogurt with the avocado mash and chicken, add lemon juice to taste. Season with kosher salt and fresh ground pepper and set aside.

VEGGIE SOUP

NUTRITION :

calories 198, Fat 5g, Carbs 31g, Protein 3g

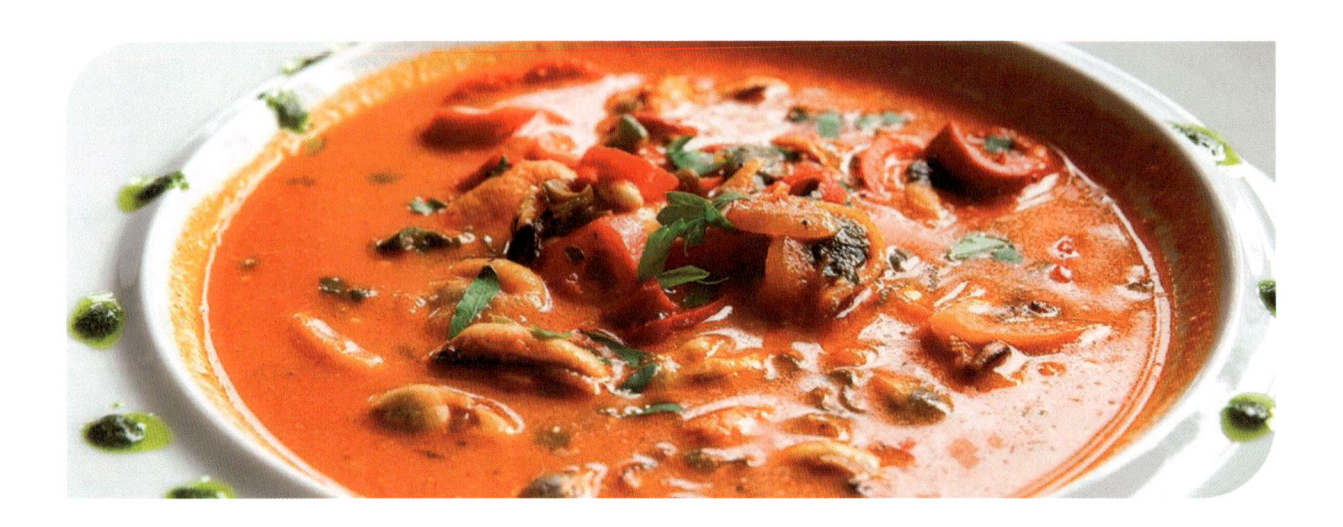

Ingredients

2 Tbsp olive oil

1/2 cups chopped yellow onion

1 cups peeled and chopped carrots (about 5)

1 cups chopped celery

4 cloves garlic , minced

1 (14.5 oz) cans low-sodium chicken broth* or vegetable broth

1 (14.5 oz) cans diced tomatoes

1 cups peeled and 1/2-inch thick diced potatoes

1/3 cup chopped fresh parsley

2 bay leaves

1/2 tsp dried thyme

Salt and freshly ground black pepper

1 1/4 cups frozen or fresh corn

1 cup frozen or fresh peas

RECIPE:

In a large stock pot, combine broth, tomato juice, water and all the ingredients. Season with salt and pepper. Bring to a boil and simmer for 30 minutes or until all vegetables are tender.

AVOCADO SALAD

NUTRITION :

126 calories; 10 g fat; 10.2 g carbohydrates; 2.1 g protein

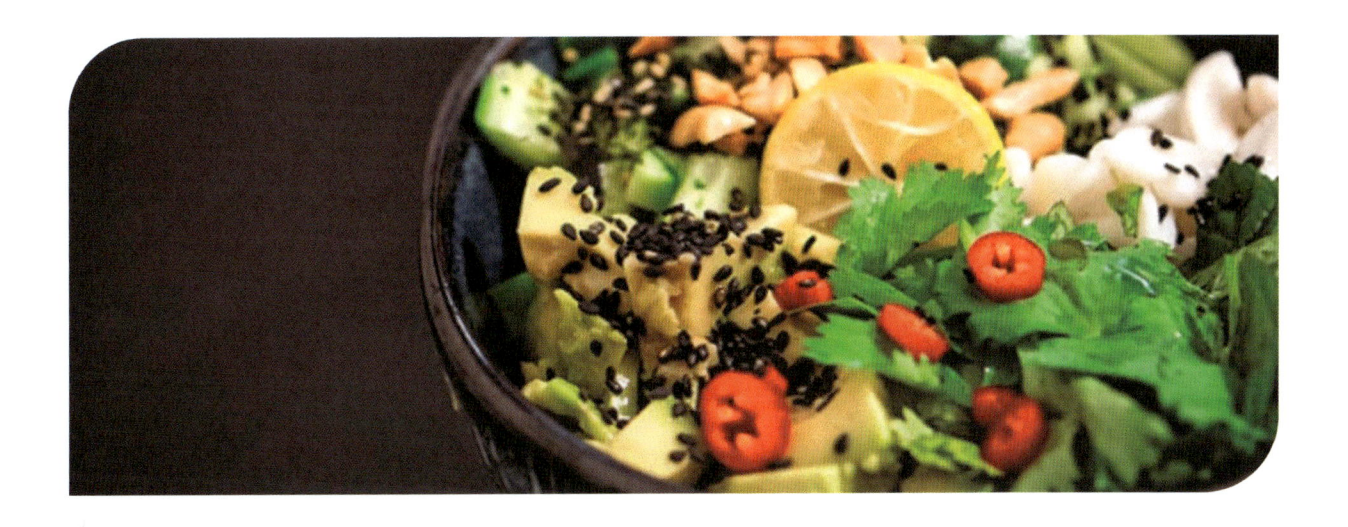

Ingredients

1 large tomato

1 English cucumber

1/2 medium red onion sliced

2 avocados diced

1 sweet onion, chopped

1 green bell pepper, chopped

1/4 cup chopped fresh cilantro

1/2 lime, juice

salt and pepper to taste

RECIPE:

1. Place chopped tomatoes, sliced cucumber, sliced red onion, diced avocado, and chopped cilantro into a large salad bowl.
2. Drizzle with 2 Tbsp lemon juice. Toss gently to combine. Just before serving, toss with sea salt and black pepper.

CHOPPED GRILLED VEGGIE SALAD

NUTRITION :

Calories 248, Fat 22g, Carbs 15g, Protein 7g

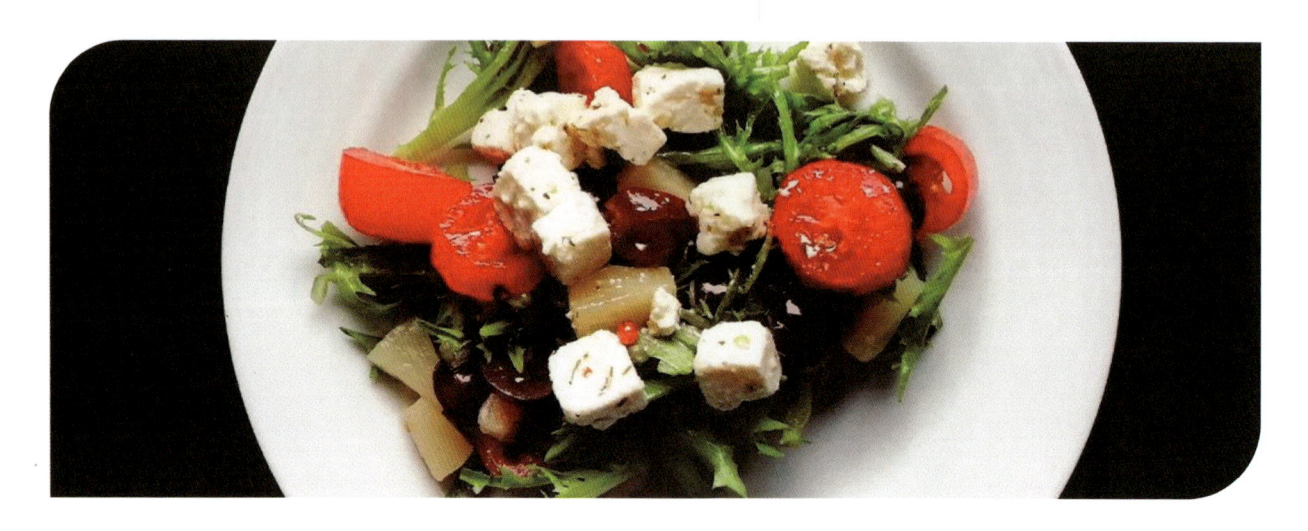

Ingredients

3 cups vegetable broth

1 portobello mushroom

1 red bell pepper seeded and quartered

8 ounces asparagus

1/2 red onion sliced

Olive oil

Kosher salt and freshly ground black pepper

1 pint plain Greek yogurt

1 clove garlic pressed

2 tablespoons minced cucumber

1 tablespoon lemon juice

1 teaspoon chopped fresh mint

1 teaspoon chopped fresh dill

Kosher salt

Red bell pepper hummus

1/8 cup feta cheese crumbled

RECIPE:

In a small bowl, mix the yogurt, garlic, cucumber, lemon juice, fresh mint and dill together. Season with salt to taste.

Chop the grilled vegetables into bite size pieces. Mix all the ingredients in a bowl and serve.

CHICKEN SPINACH SALAD

NUTRITION :

Calories 178kcal, Fat 8g, Carbs 11g, Protein 16g

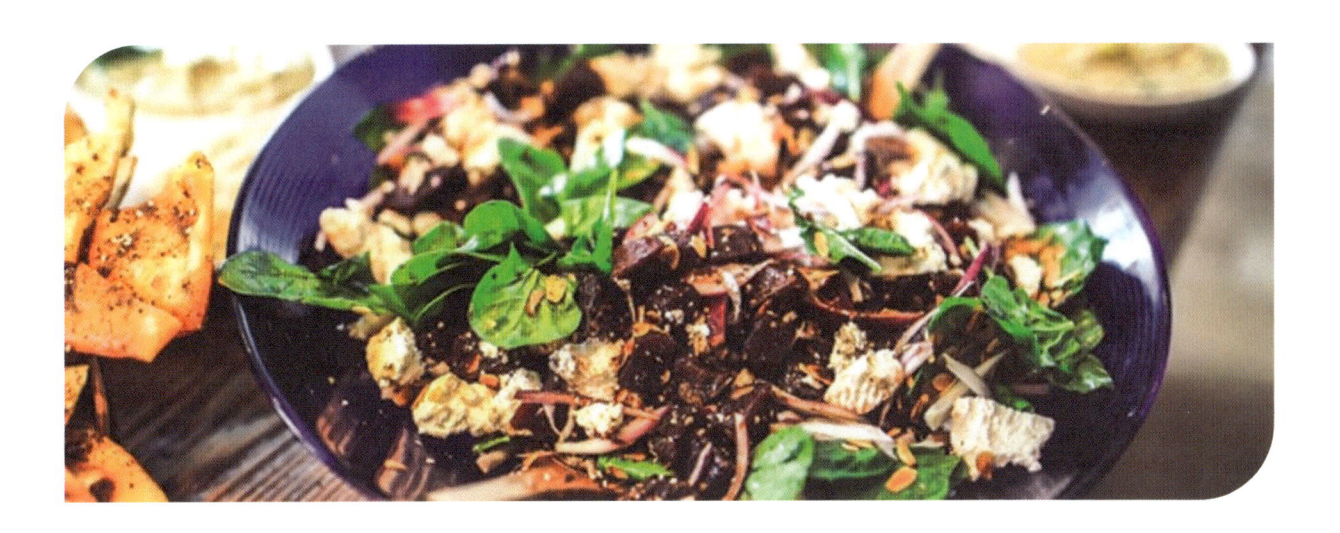

Ingredients

4 fillets Grilled chicken

7 oz bag baby spinach

½ sweet red bell pepper

1 cup grape tomatoes, halved

1 carrot, sliced

Red onion, thinly sliced

1 tbsp. lemon juice

RECIPE:

1. Combine all the ingredients in a medium bowl.
2. Cut the chicken into slices and add into the bowl with spinach and other ingredients.
3. Sprinkle some lemon juice and serve.

GROCERY LIST WEEK 4

Whole-grain bread	Pepperoni	4 12oz salmon fillets	Brown rice	Red onions	Baking potatoes	Mozzarella cheese
Peanut butter	Mozzarella cheese	Soy sauce	Tomatoes	Avocados	Cilantro	Vegetable oil
Bananas	Butter	Salt	Black Pepper	Sweet onions	Lemons	
Icing sugar	Dipping sauce	Garlic powder	Cucumbers	Green bell pepper	2 cans baked beans	Cream cheese
Almond flour	Italian seasoning	Baking powder	Unsweetened tomato sauce	Dried oregano	Pepperoni	Olives
2 can chickpeas	Spinach	Feta cheese	Raisins	Honey	Cumin	Chili flakes
Canola oil	Maple syrup	Strawberries	Basil	Mixed berries	Hummus	Celery

MEAL PLAN WEEK 4

DAY	BREAKFAST	LUNCH	DINNER	SNACKS
MONDAY	Boiled egg with mayonnaise	Grilled salmon with brown rice	Chickpea spinach salad	3 carrots with a half cup of hummus
TUESDAY	Pizza rollups	Avocado salad	Baked salmon	2 hard-boiled eggs
WEDNESDAY	Peanut butter banana toast	Grilled salmon with brown rice	Strawberry & basil salad	5 celery sticks and peanut butter
THURSDSAY	Pizza rollups	Baked potato & beans	Chickpea spinach salad	Cup of berries
FRIDAY	Peanut butter banana toast	Instant pizza	Baked salmon	Bowl of sliced cucumbers
SATURDAY	Boiled egg with mayonnaise	Baked potato & beans	Strawberry & basil salad	3 carrots with a half cup of hummus
SUNDAY	Strawberry smoothie	Avocado salad	Chicken soup	Hard-boiled egg An apple

PIZZA ROLL UPS

NUTRITION :

Calories: 75, Total Carbohydrates: 0g, Fat: 5g, Protein: 8g

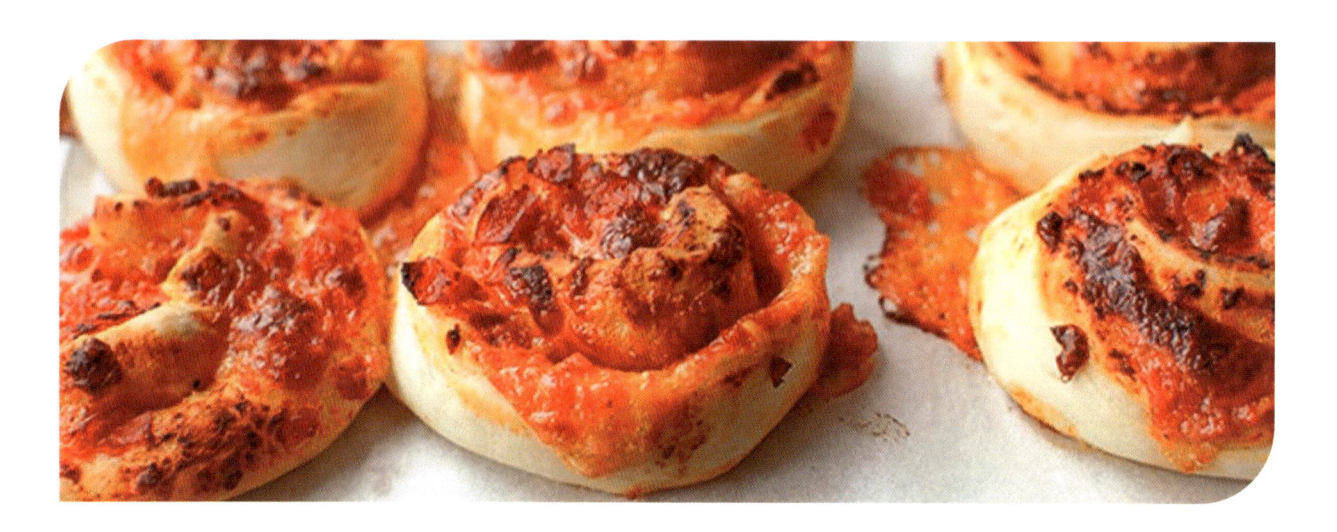

Ingredients

8 oz. cheddar cheese
2 oz. butter
Mini pepperoni slices
Dipping sauce

RECIPE:

1. Place the cheese slices on a large cutting board.
2. Cut really thin pieces of butter with a knife.
3. Add as little or as much pepperoni as you would like.
4. Gently roll them up and serve.

GRILLED SALMON WITH BROWN RICE

NUTRITION :

Calories 318, Fat 20g, Carbs 12g, Protein 20g

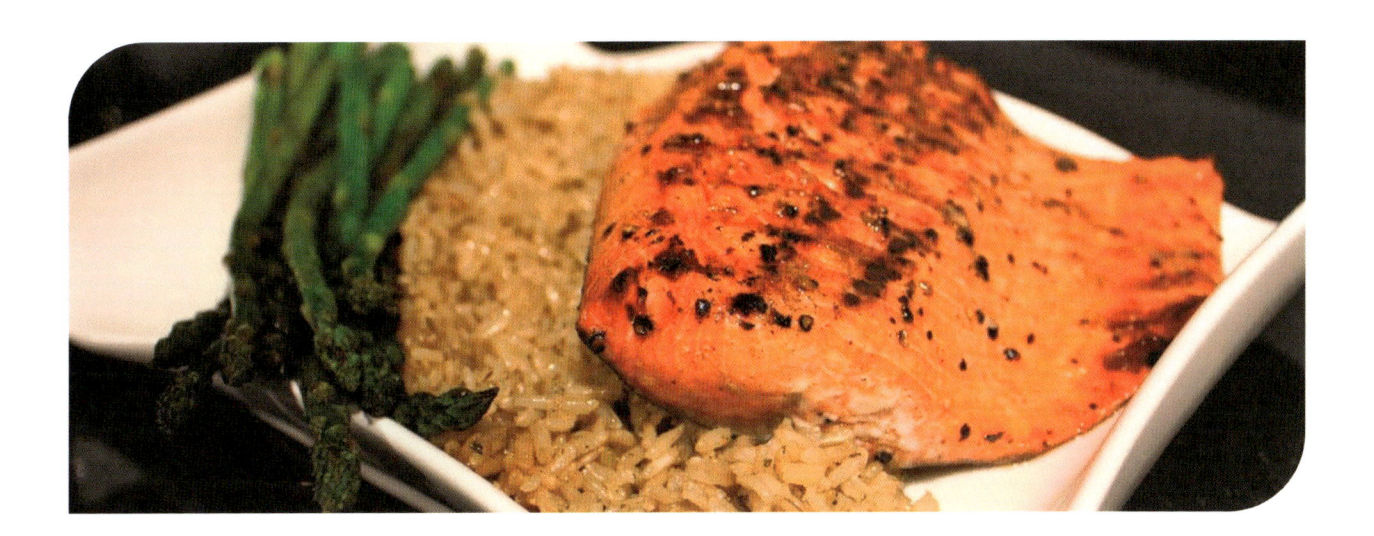

Ingredients

12 Oz salmon fillet
Salt
Black pepper
1/3 cup Soy sauce
Garlic powder
1 cup Brown rice
Water

RECIPE:

1. Preheat grill for medium heat.
2. Coat the salmon fillets with oil, salt, black pepper, garlic powder and soy sauce.
3. Place the fillet on the grill and cook for 6-8 minutes or until the salmon is golden brown and flaky.
4. Change the side and repeat the step.
5. Serve with brown rice

FOR BROWN RICE :

1. Add 6 cups of water and a pinch of salt into a large pot and place it over the heat to boil.
2. Rinse the rice under running water
3. Add the rice into the boiling water
4. Adjust the temperature reduce accordingly.
5. Boil it for at least 25-30 minutes or until soft uncovered .
6. drain the water from the rice and shift the rice back to the pot and let it rest for 5-10 minutes.

BAKED POTATO & BEANS

NUTRITION :

Calories 120 kcal, Fat 2g, Carbs 18g, Protein 5g

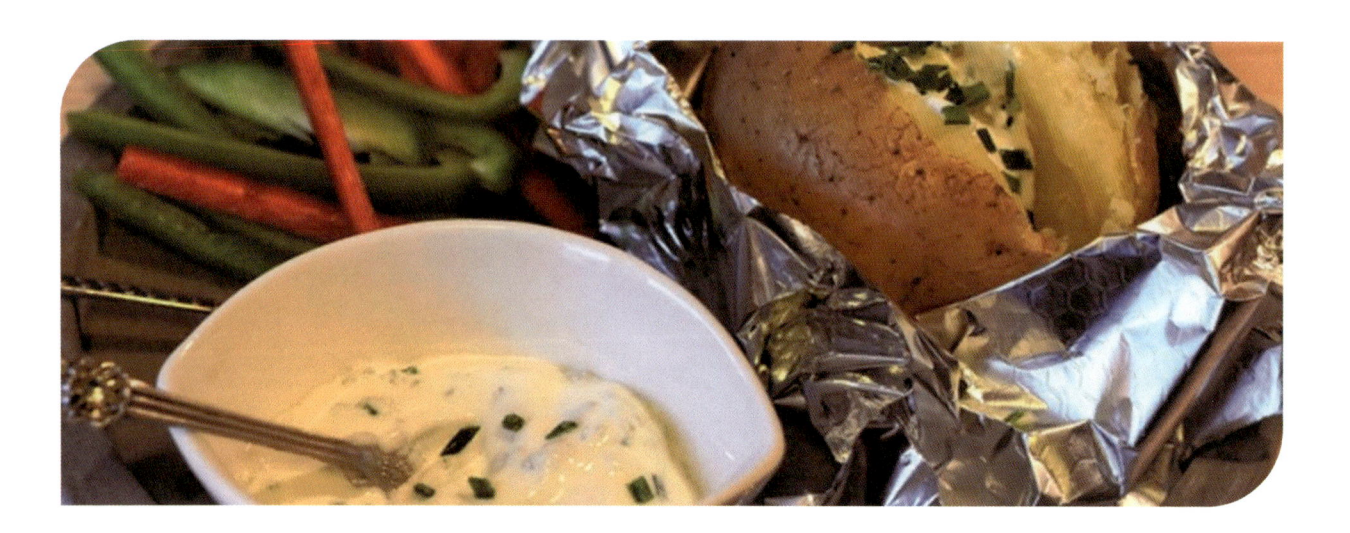

Ingredients

4 baking potatoes

2 cans baked beans (reduced sugar)

Cheddar cheese/ mozzarella cheese

4 tbsp. olive oil/vegetable oil

RECIPE:

1. Set the oven to 400F. wash and prick the potatoes with a fork.
2. Cover each potato in a teaspoon of oil.
3. Place the potatoes in preheated oven and bake for almost 90 minutes or until slightly soft or golden brown.
4. Gently heat the beans in the pan for about 3-5 minutes until hot, stirring continuously .
5. Slice the potato from the center and spoon grated cheese and beans in the potato.

INSTANT PIZZA

NUTRITION:

Calories: 249kcal, Carbohydrates: 5g, Protein: 14g, Fat: 19g

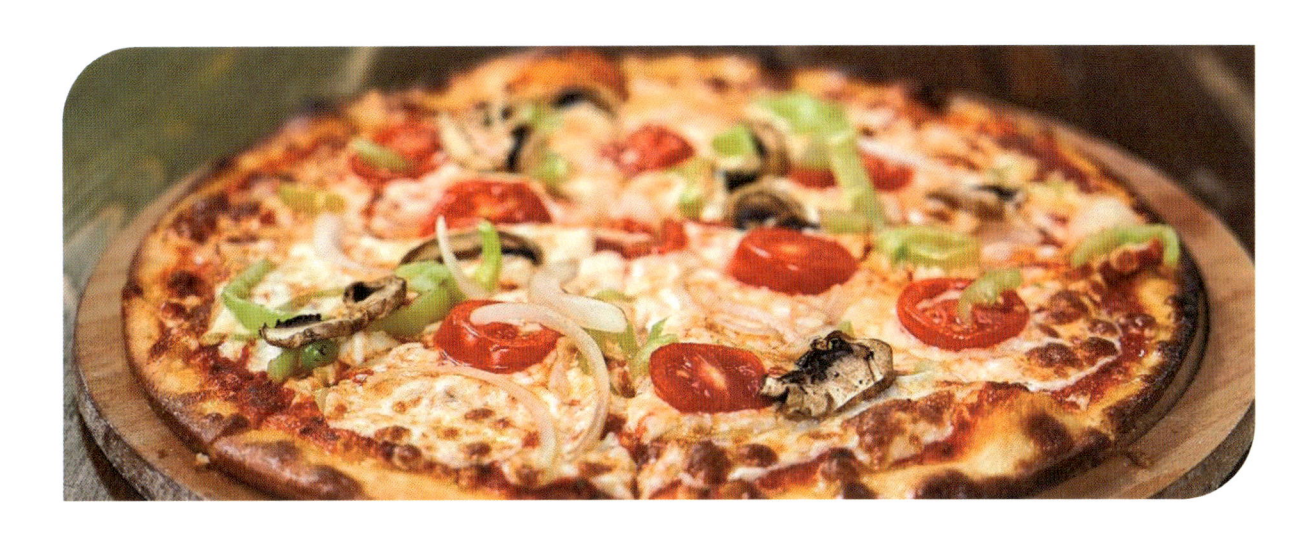

Ingredients

2 cups Shredded Mozzarella Cheese

1 oz cream cheese

1 cup Almond flour

1 egg

1 teaspoon baking powder

1 teaspoon Italian seasoning

TOPPINGS

3 tbsp unsweetened tomato sauce

1 tsp dried oregano

5 oz. shredded cheese

1½ oz. pepperoni

olives

RECIPE:

1. Pre-heat oven to 450F.
2. Add mozzarella and cream cheese to a large microwave-safe bowl and microwave for 45 seconds.
3. Remove from microwave and add in egg, almond flour, baking powder, Italian seasoning, and garlic. Mix with a spoon.
4. Transfer dough onto a baking sheet lined with parchment paper.
5. Make a round and bake in the oven for 12-15 minutes until the crust turns golden.
6. Remove from oven and add toppings like sauces, cheese, and other toppings.
7. Bake pizza for another 6-10 minutes or until it turns golden brown.

CHICKPEA SPINACH SALAD

NUTRITION :

Calories 680, Fat 40g, Carbs 52g, Protein 23g

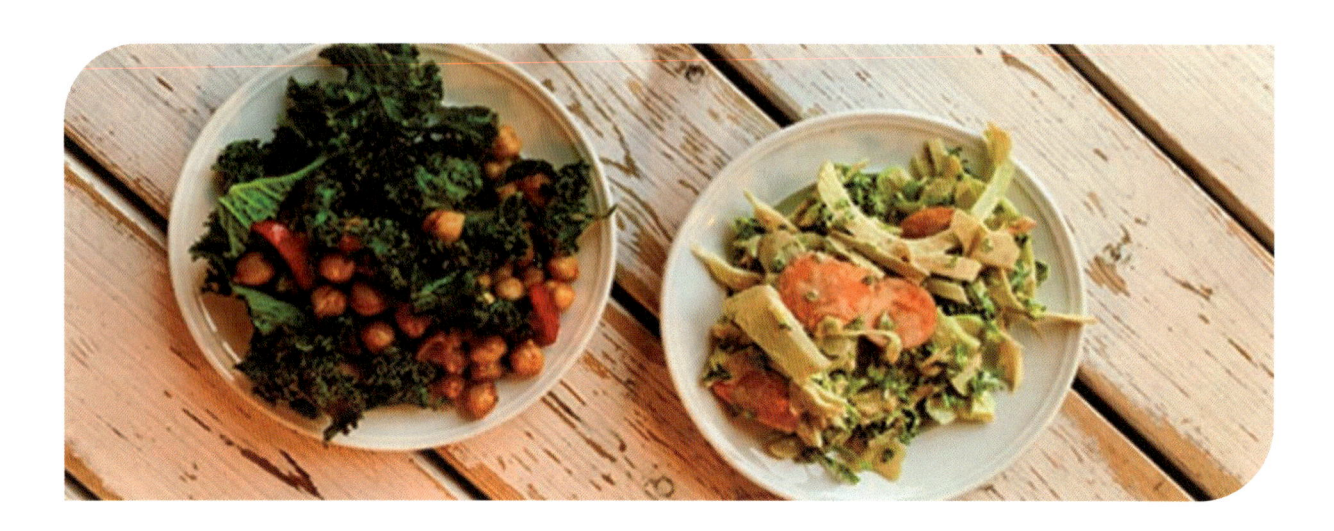

Ingredients

1 can chickpeas (drained and rinsed)
1 handful spinach
3.5 oz feta cheese
1 small handful raisins
½ tbsp lemon juice
3 tsp honey
4 tbsp olive oil
1 tsp cumin
1 pinch salt
½ tsp chili flakes

RECIPE:

1. Chop the cheese and add with the spinach and chickpeas to a large bowl.
2. Mix the honey, oil, lemon juice and raisins in a small bowl.
3. Add the cumin, salt and pepper to the dressing bowl and mix well.
4. Drizzle devilishly delicious dressing over the salad.

BAKED SALMON

NUTRITION :

Calories 170, Fat 11g, Carbs 0g, Protein 15g

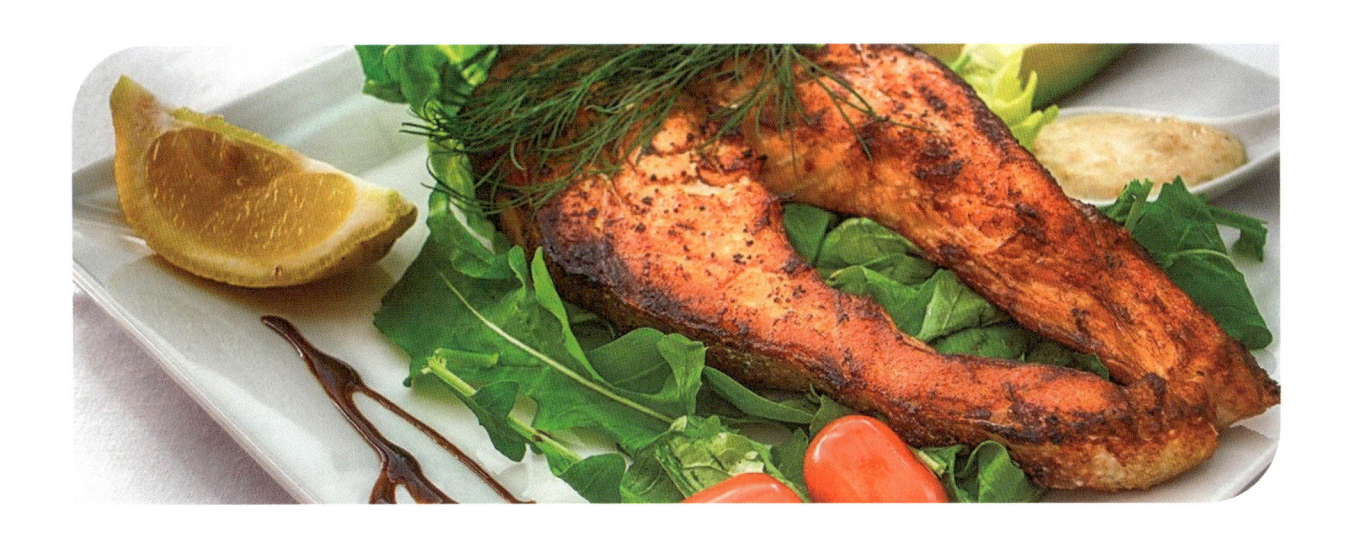

Ingredients

12 oz salmon fillet
Salt
Black pepper
2 tbsp. canola oil

RECIPE:

1. Preheat the oven to 450F.
2. Place the salmon fillet on the non-stick pan or baking sheet with aluminum foil.
3. Brush the salmon with oil except for bottom area and sprinkle with black pepper and salt.
4. Bake until the salmon is cooked enough for about 10-15 minutes.
5. Serve with the sauce of your choice.

Printed in Great Britain
by Amazon